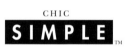

CHIC
SIMPLE ™

DO YOU DRESS SMART™?

You only have seven seconds to make an impression. Clothes make the difference—dress smart.

1. I work for a traditional law firm with a strict corporate dress code. I am traveling with my boss to a three-day conference that we leave for on a Sunday afternoon. Can I wear my weekend jeans and sneakers on our flight? ....YES or NO

2. Do I need to wear a suit to my interview if I know the office dresses casual? ....YES or NO

3. I don't see my upper management very often, so is there any point in making an investment in my business wardrobe? ....YES or NO

4. I am an accountant at a firm that employs a corporate dress code. I have a meeting at a client's firm that has a casual dress code. Should I follow their dress code for the meeting? ....YES or NO

5. Throughout college and summer jobs I have always worn loafers without socks—would that be appropriate on casual Fridays in the summer? ....YES or NO

6. I am forty years old in a youth-oriented company, and I'm in competition for a promotion. Should I update my image with a more hip look (i.e., younger)? ....YES or NO

7. I think my boss dresses too casually for his position. Is it okay for me to dress more formally than him? ....YES or NO

8. Can I wear a button-down shirt with a pinstripe suit? ....YES or NO

9. I just got a promotion where I now oversee an entire department. A suit is just a suit whether I pay $ or $$$, so do I need to change my wardrobe? ....YES or NO

10. I believe I should be judged by the work I do and not the way I look. Does it really make a difference to "dress the part," if my work is good? ....YES or NO

1. no 2. yes 3. yes 4. no 5. no 6. no 7. yes 8. yes 9. yes 10. yes

DRESS SMART™ MEN

Wardrobes That Win in the New Workplace

Kim Johnson Gross and Jeff Stone
Text by Michael Solomon
Photos by David Bashaw

WARNER BOOKS

NEW YORK   BOSTON

Text by Michael Solomon
Photographs by David Bashaw
Set Stylist Renee Yan
Editorial Consultant Matthew Mol

Warner Books

Time Warner Book Group
1271 Avenue of the Americas, New York, NY 10020
Visit Chic Simple at www.twbookmark.com

Printed in England
First Edition: September 2002
10   9   8   7   6   5   4   3   2

Library of Congress Cataloging-in-Publication Data
Gross, Kim Johnson.
Dress Smart—men : wardrobes that win in the new workplace / Kim Johnson Gross and Jeff Stone ;
text by Michael Solomon ; photos by David Bashaw.
p.cm. — (Chic Simple)
Includes index.
ISBN 0-446-53043-3
1. Men's clothing. 2. Grooming for men. I. Stone, Jeff, 1953– II. Solomon, Michael, 1966– III. Title. IV. Series.
TT618.G7597 2002
646'.32—dc21

2002025897

Separations by Butler & Tanner Limited

CHIC SIMPLE is a primer for living well but sensibly. It's for those who believe that quality of life comes not from accumulating things but in paring down to the essentials. Chic Simple enables readers to bring value and style into their lives with economy and simplicity.

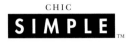

"It is possible through the skillful manipulation of dress in any particular situation to evoke a favorable response to your positioning and your needs."

JOHN T. MOLLOY
New Dress for Success

Dear Reader,

To paraphrase John T. Molloy—people do judge a book by its cover. Right or wrong, it's just the real world. Dressing appropriately in today's workplace is essential. Your clothes are the first impression you make whether on a job interview, representing your firm to a new client, or making a presentation within your company. Bottom line: You should always dress for the job you want, and for your professional goals.

But today the simple act of dressing can be confusing. Mistakes can be costly not only to your budget, but also to your career. *Dress Smart*™ offers practical guidelines and sound, simple advice to help you determine your best professional wardrobe.

This book has been culled from our own experience as consultants working with a variety of companies who made the transition from corporate-wear to casual Friday and are now moving to a blend of the two worlds. These observations have been reinforced by the countless e-mails we receive daily on the Chic Simple web site (www.chicsimple.com), from men around the country who are confused about real work-wear questions.

We feel that the two *Dress Smart*™ books (we've also written a companion to this book, *Dress Smart*™ *Women*) are the most important of the 25 Chic Simple titles we have published over the last 10 years. Why? Because *Dress Smart*™ will give you the confidence that accompanies dressing appropriately and with authority. Whether you want to get a job, be a success at your present job or get a better job—*Dress Smart*™ is the first crucial step because small investments in your wardrobe lead to large payoffs in your career. Don't hesitate to invest in yourself.

Now go get dressed.

jeff and Kim

"The more you know, the less you need."
AUSTRALIAN ABORIGINAL SAYING

HOW TO use this book

It's broken into the three major aspects of your work life/career:

1. GET JOB (hard to work without one)
2. SUCCEED IN JOB (good idea)
3. GET BETTER JOB (better is better)

At each stage, *Dress Smart*™ reviews the issues you should be aware of, concrete ways to convert these ideas into clothes, and examples of how to work those clothes into everyday life. We use the **image guides** to do the translating; each critical stage ends with a sample closet.

1. GET JOB.

If you are leaving college and going into the job market, if you are reentering the job market after a sabbatical, or if you just decided to get serious about the whole job/career thing and want to shoot for something different, then focus on section one. The principles are the same no matter what stage you're at.

2. SUCCEED IN JOB.

You've decided that work is a significant part of your life, you are serious about taking it to the next stage, and you want to never worry about looking appropriate no matter the moment or opportunity—your clothes should be a secret asset.

3. GET BETTER JOB.

Today more people than ever are competing for the top jobs. Congratulations, you pulled it off—but do you look it? Here's the skinny on looking the part, even if you'd rather be sailing off Baja or kayaking in Chile—at least your clothes won't give you away. It's easy: turn the pages, read, look, and think about what you want your clothes to say about you.

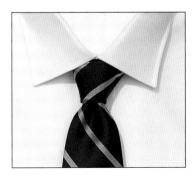 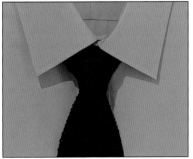 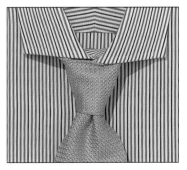

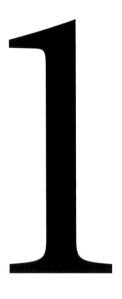

GET JOB

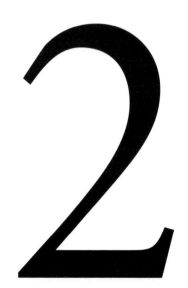

SUCCEED IN JOB

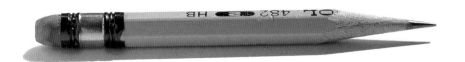

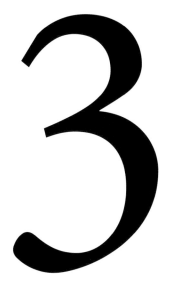

3

GET BETTER JOB

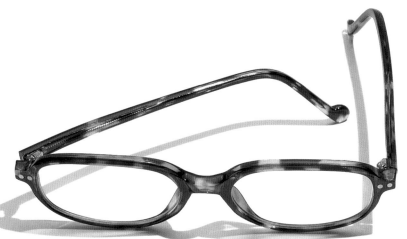

4

GOES WITH THE JOB

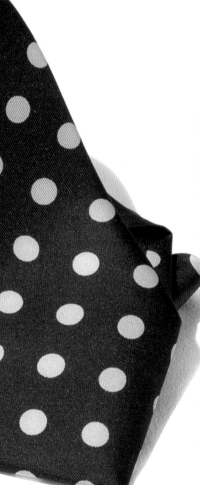

FIT TO BE TIED

Dear jeff and Kim,
My girlfriend feels that it looks sophisticated to wear a shirt and sweater to a job interview. She feels the "suit image" is fake. I'm nervous. I don't want to blow my chances, but I don't want to look like I'm trying too hard either. Most of the people I know doing this type of work (communications) dress casually in the office. So is a tie and suit too old-fashioned?
—Tie Shy

Dear Tie Shy,
Feeling nervous is normal. Jobs are not easy to land. You are probably interviewing with the HR manager, who expects to see you looking your best (maybe he never will again). It's packaging, packaging, packaging. You are trying to show that you know how to present yourself in a work environment. Keep it simple: White or blue shirt, simple tie, dark suit. Wear the "sophisticated outfit" when you go out with your girlfriend to celebrate getting the job.

—jeff and Kim

Get Job 1

Interview Wardrobe

Seconds… tick, tick, tick, tick… *Mission Impossible* seconds are counting down as the HR manager stretches out a hand and BANG! You are registered, judged, and mentally filed away. So what's on that file? Have you set up the groundwork for a smooth interview and job offer, or a wary "we'll see what's here," or "what a bozo—when can I get rid of this guy?" This section is about putting together the most winning combination of visual reinforcements and clues, so you can make a positive impression on your interviewer. Bottom line—you're reading this because you want a job. Help yourself get that job. Read on.

1. Get Job

If You're So Smart, Why Do You Dress So Stupid?
—Clothes & Career

DRESSING THE PART

In 1912, the New York Highlanders took the baseball field in what would become the most famous uniform in sports history: Pinstripes. By the 1930s, the pattern on their uniform had come to define the first power look for men. As orderly as the lines on a banker's ledger, the pinstripe suit signified a man's stature in the corporate world. Meanwhile, the New York Yankees (as the Highlanders were now known) had become the most dominant team in the major leagues, and their pinstripes had already taken on a mystique: Did Yankees owner Col. Jacob Ruppert really insist on the uniforms just to make Babe Ruth look slimmer? Or perhaps the message was even simpler: In pinstripes, the Yankees were all business.

Today, whether it's baseball or banking, how a man dresses can affect not only his performance, but also his career itself. If you don't present yourself properly on a job interview, you may not get in the door. Once inside, you need to look the part to stay there and move up. And eventually, if you want to move high up or out, you need to be aware of the messages you are sending others.

THE POWER OF IMAGE

Consider the paintings of the Impressionist Georges Seurat: From far away, they are seemingly of an idyllic Sunday afternoon by the lake or a day at the Eiffel Tower. But move closer and you see that Seurat's images are, in fact, tiny dots of color. His pointillist style is actually nothing more than perfectly positioned brush strokes, which, when viewed as a whole, produce the big picture.

Dressing smart requires the same thinking: How you put all of the elements of your wardrobe together can either create an image that is visually pleasing or something that's a big mess. In order to understand whether you are in fact an artist like Seurat, you have to break down the elements of your appearance dot by dot. Does your suit frame your body well? Is that tie too distracting? Are your shoes tripping people up? By examining each aspect of your wardrobe you can develop the style that best suits who you are and eventually use that style to set yourself apart.

STYLE AND SUBSTANCE

How a man dresses and looks is obviously important, but what defines his style? The people we often consider the best dressed do not typically wear clothing we remember. There is not usually one item that stands out on such a man, he merely seems to put everything together well and carries himself with great sophistication. He is well groomed; his hair, nails, and general appearance seem clean and polished (as are his shoes).

His style is often defined by confidence, which some are born with and others acquire over time. It is a confidence not simply in what he is wearing, but rather in who he is. In other words, style without substance is meaningless. A great shirt and tie might help you get a job, but they will never do the work for you. Without the talent and drive to back up the promise of your appearance, you are merely an empty suit.

THE TREND GAME

Fashion is a scary word for men—and for good reason. It is mostly concerned with trends—wearing the clothes that will be appropriate for one season, and perhaps not even that long. The world of fashion is obsessed with name-brand designers and labels that will impress a small section of society. There is nothing wrong with wanting to be fashionable, of course. But as with the best things in life, following trends is best enjoyed in moderation: A bold shirt, a graphic tie, an eye-catching pair of cuff links.

Style, on the other hand, is timeless. A blue blazer, gray flannels,

"Let us be thankful for the fools; but for them the rest of us could not succeed."

MARK TWAIN

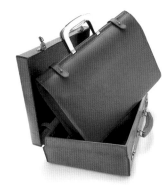

loafers, these items are considered classics for a reason: They will never go out of style and will never be inappropriate. When building a wardrobe for work, it is always better to err on the side of classic. After all, if you intend to be on the job for several years, shouldn't you expect the same of your clothing?

DRESSING (SMART) FOR SUCCESS

In 1975, John T. Molloy published his now classic book, *Dress for Success*. At the time, there was nothing like it to guide a man through the principles of proper attire in the workplace, and his sartorial homilies taught a generation how to "dress like a million so you can make a million." Molloy's philosophy was relatively simple: Clothing affects business performance and influences the way superiors and peers view you. And, playing to our most basic "keeping up with the Joneses" mentality, Molloy argues that even if you don't want to dress to get ahead, the next guy will.

Over the years, much of Molloy's advice still held true, but the workplace changed dramatically in the past quarter century. Molloy never foresaw the advent of casual Fridays and corporate policies that allowed for khakis and polo shirts in the office. How exactly were you supposed to dress for a meeting with 20-something dot-com millionaires who were wearing ripped jeans and T-shirts?

Today, however, the economy has shifted yet again, and the days of casual dressing in the office have waned. As corporate belts have tightened, employees are paying more attention to their pants—and suits and ties. Work has once again become business as usual, but what does business look like?

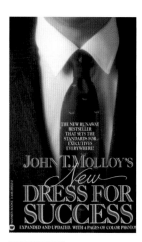

THANK YOU, JOHN MOLLOY

An important feature of Molloy's book was the testing of his theories about clothes and how people react to them. He would test everyone from receptionists to doormen to maître d's. And by recruiting variously dressed individuals in different outfits and color combinations he was able to deduce the power of suits, raincoats, and shirt-and-tie combinations. It proved that appearances count—especially to receptionists.

Clothes Talk, People Listen

"We'd all
like to be
taken for
what we'd
like to be."
MALCOLM FORBES

In the high-tech, high-speed world we live in, instant gratification is often not soon enough. We like our news 24 hours a day and expect tomorrow's information to be here yesterday. Among the many perils of this fast-paced society is that we are quick to make judgments about the appearances of others. In such a world, we need to send signals immediately and hope that people get the message we intend to send.

When Steve Case, chairman of America Online, and Gerald Levin, chairman of Time Warner, announced the merger of their two companies, their clothing generated nearly as much news as their business deal. Case, the epitome of a laid-back dot-com mogul, appeared at the press conference in a tie, while Levin, a lifelong corporate soldier, chose not to wear one. Of course, at the CEO level, one can, for the most part, dress as one chooses, but such a public fashion statement sent a clear signal that the two corporate worlds had already begun to blend.

CLOTHES-MINDED

So what are your clothes saying about you? It's not always easy to know because, like having bad breath or spinach in your teeth, people are not likely to tell you when you are dressed inappropriately. The goal is to determine the ultimate message you want to send. And for the most part, that message is simple: You want to appear competent at all times and show people that you belong.

1. Get Job

Each office, whether it's a white-shoe law firm or a red-hot advertising agency, has a dress code. Adhere to it and you signal to everyone that you are part of the team. This is not to say that individuality can't be expressed, but sometimes the best impression is no impression at all. In other words, you dress so appropriately for the office that no one notices. It is simply assumed that you always look the part.

Of course, adhering to the clothing standards of an office or industry does not guarantee that you will make a good impression. Imagine that two junior salesmen with very similar skill sets are up for the same promotion at an insurance company where the men all wear suits or sport jackets and most wear ties. One of the candidates always dresses in a sport jacket, crisp white shirts, and creased trousers, but he never wears a tie. The other always wears a suit and tie to the office, but his shirts are usually wrinkled, his ties are frequently stained, and his shoes look as though they haven't been shined since he bought them. Who gets the job? Well, the first guy may never wear a tie, but he clearly pays attention to other clothing details, and others will relate that to his work ethic. He looks sharp and ready for action and eventually, perhaps from the money he'll get from the promotion, he'll get himself a few ties.

The lesson here is that dressing smart is not always about dressing formally. Paying attention to the subtleties of style may impact your appearance far more than simply adhering to an overall dress code.

DRESSING AS IF YOUR (PROFESSIONAL) LIFE DEPENDED ON IT

In today's business environment, there are more potentially hazardous clothing situations than ever—breakfast meetings, client lunches, black-tie dinners, golf outings, board presentations, TV appearances—and dressing smart means you have to be prepared for every one of them. Clearly, you cannot wear the same outfit for all of those occasions, but you can maintain a certain standard that suggests you could be ready for any one of them at a moment's notice. For instance, a coworker calls in sick and can't make it to a charity dinner that night. Your boss mentally runs through replacement options. He knows that you come to work in a suit every day, so he asks if you have a tuxedo. You do, of course, and suddenly you become the tenth person at the table—seated two places away from the CEO.

How to Dress Smart™
—The Chic Simple Process

ASSESS, DEJUNK, RENEW—UNDERSTANDING THE CHIC SIMPLE PROCESS

Building the perfect work wardrobe does not happen by accident. You could go to work for a decade and not have a proper wardrobe because you didn't identify your needs carefully enough. You could have built one in several years, but, because you didn't take care of your clothes properly, they are actually working against you. Or perhaps you simply have a wardrobe that is outdated.

The key to an ideal work wardrobe can be explained in three easy steps:

1. ASSESS: YOUR LIFE, YOUR CLOSET

When you are finally ready to be serious about your professional life, you have to accept this reality: All the clothes you normally wear are play clothes. Sure, you may get compliments on them and they might even look fine in a nice restaurant, but your career is serious business and you should now understand that you must have work clothes to match.

The first step in assessing your clothing needs is to recognize that your closet is like your desk. The better organized your desk is, the easier it is to find that stapler you need. The same is true for shirts and ties, shoes and suits. Arrange your closet by work and play, week and weekend. The suits stay with the sport jackets, the jeans and khakis are

1. Get Job

arranged with each other. Your dress shirts (especially the white ones) should be easily delineated from the casual shirts you wear on Saturdays. Sneakers don't mix with dress shoes, and so on. With a little bit of work your closet will be ready for work.

2. DEJUNK: TAKING INVENTORY

Now that your closet is neatly arranged, what do you have in there? Are there clothes you haven't worn in a year or so? Get rid of them. Are there sport jackets that are too big? Take them to the tailor. Pants that are two sizes too small? Give them to a thinner friend. Ties with soup stains? Let the dry cleaner hit the spot. Shoes with holes in them? Walk away.

Now is the time to make room in your closet using the triage method. And if you just can't decide if something you own should be tossed, here's a smart standard: Would you want to see yourself wearing it in a picture ten years from now? If not, let it go.

3. RENEW: SHOPPING YOUR CLOSET

Once you've removed the unnecessary (or offending) items, look to see what's missing. Do you have enough shirts, but too few ties? Plenty of pants, but only one pair of shoes? No black socks?

The best way to determine your needs is to make a list. In one column, list all the things in your closet. In the column next to it, name all the clothing that would make that item more versatile (Left: Black-and-white houndstooth jacket. Right: White shirt, black tie, gray pants, black pants, black shoes, gray polo sweater). The right-hand side will then become your shopping list. And if there are items on the list that can go with several other things in your closet (such as the gray trousers), then circle those items and make them a priority when shopping. The more versatile the purchase, the smarter the shopper.

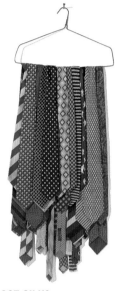

GOT SILK?
Too overwhelmed to deal with your closet? Start small. Look at your collection of ties—the gifts, the mistakes (it's okay, Jerry Garcia never wore his ties either)—and start to divide into recycle and keepers. Next week take the keeper pile and do it again.

1. Assess

Assess and survey. Take account of how you live your life and what you own. These are the key two areas of examination you need to engage in. Match your possessions with your life and voilà—your focus returns.

A PROCESS OF SIMPLICITY

2. DeJunk

DeJunk and recycle. Simplify is a verb, a practice. You must act, deal with all that is superfluous, think hard about what you actually need, and edit ruthlessly. In the end, it will save you grief, time, and money.

3. ReNew

ReNew and replace. You thought about what you need, you got rid of what you didn't need, and now it's time to fill in the holes. Does this mean shopping or rethinking? Learn how you can prevent repeating mistakes.

Cracking the Dress Codes of Business

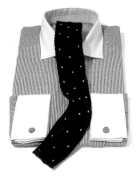

CORPORATE
Tie constant.

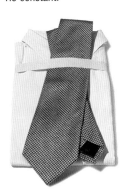

BUSINESS APPROPRIATE
Tie optional.

FOUR DRESS CODES OF BUSINESS

Company dress codes are not well defined and are rarely written down. They are mostly gleaned by observing: "What are my peers wearing? How do my superiors dress?" etc. But there are three basic dress codes that every office usually falls into, as well as one personal dress code. Follow these guidelines and you will be safe.

CORPORATE DRESS CODE

The most formal standard of dress there is, the corporate dress code means suits with shirts (usually white) and ties. This is the dress code of law firms and investment banks. In the past few years, the corporate dress code has eased somewhat, but it is recently coming back strong. Once again, the "suits" upstairs are wearing suits.

BUSINESS CASUAL DRESS CODE

If every day were casual Friday, this is the dress code that would apply. In the business casual world, not only is a suit not necessary, but a jacket may not even be required. But a casual dress code does not mean that you can let it all hang out. In fact, neatness may count more than ever in this environment. If you wear khakis and a white oxford shirt to work most days, make sure they're clean and pressed. Polish your shoes and never wear sneakers to the office. Wear sweaters that fit well and not ones that are baggy, wrinkled, or have holes in them. A sense of professionalism must be maintained at all times.

THE EVOLUTION OF BUSINESS APPROPRIATE

Business has often been cast as a Darwinian struggle, and the development of business appropriate dress in the workplace is an excellent example of the phenomena. Over the past 20 years the pendulum of corporate dress has swung from one extreme to the other: Starting with the buttoned-up world of pinstripes and power ties to the worn-down world of faded jeans and T-shirts. CEOs of powerful industries established both trends. In the go-go days of the Wall Street–tech bubble it became practically mandatory to dress casually to establish your credentials.

Then the bubble burst, and as the economy changed so did the dress landscape. A new dress code evolved, not from the top down but instead led by the people on the job. Without a memo in sight, people started to upgrade their look—jackets with nice dress shirts and slacks, and even an occasional tie. There's a tacit evolutionary understanding that as the times get tougher, the smart species survives by adapting to the environment.

And so business appropriate has emerged as midpoint between business casual and corporate dress codes. Silicon valley meets the man in the gray flannel suit, and business appropriate is the offspring.

BUSINESS APPROPRIATE AND BUSINESS APPROPRIATE CASUAL DRESS CODE

This dress code is somewhere between corporate and casual, and can, in some ways, be the most difficult to navigate. The business appropriate dress code requires that you have a secure sense of what is appropriate for your office and industry. A suit is no longer mandatory, but if you wear one perhaps you don't put on a tie with a dress shirt. A sport jacket and trousers with a dress shirt would also be an acceptable alternative. In the business appropriate world, one can even opt to wear a nice polo shirt or sweater with a sport jacket. The idea is that you can allow yourself some comfort, but you must always look polished and professional.

"We don't live in a world of reality, we live in a world of perceptions."

GERALD J. SIMMONS

The Evolution

Corporate

Casual

SUIT
mandatory

**SHIRT
AND TIE**
mandatory

**JACKET:
WITH TEE**
mandatory
**WITH SHIRT
OR SWEATER**
optional

JEANS
only okay if
you're the
boss or the
office is home

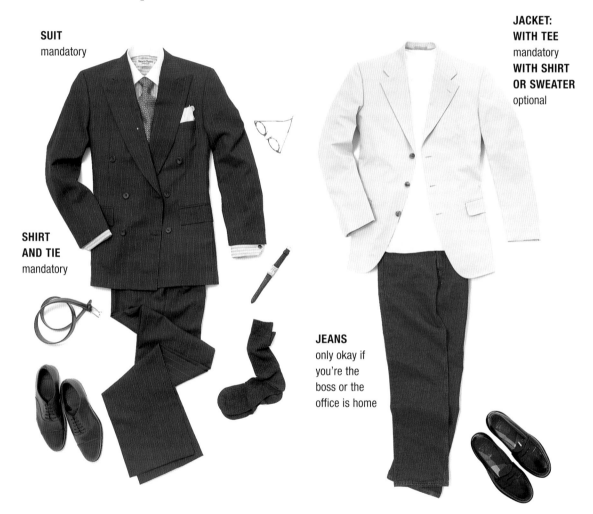

The suit and tie ensemble is a constant. A classic of American business, it has grown from a stiff authoritative structure to a more comfortable expression of business. But don't be confused. It is still about joining the club.

The days of "whatever, I'm too busy" or "too creative to bother about what I'm wearing" are over. Casual means pulled together, nothing faded or ragged. In many ways it's difficult to pull off without appearing to be trapped at summer camp.

# of Dress Codes

Business Appropriate

Business Appropriate Casual

SHIRT
mandatory
TIE
optional

SHIRT OR SWEATER
mandatory

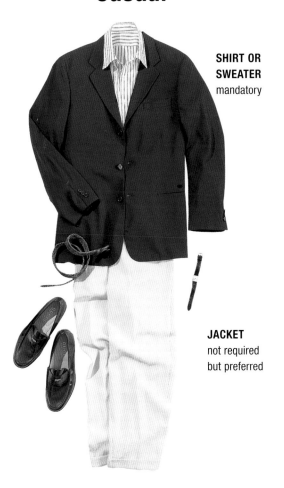

JACKET
mandatory
SUIT
preferred

JACKET
not required
but preferred

Rapidly becoming the "new standard," it is more about dressing for the context of the day or occasion—to tie or not to tie is the question. But there is a covert understanding that a jacket is a necessity.

"Casual" under this dress code means understanding that a more relaxed look is not an excuse to look like you came into work during the weekend. A good rule of thumb is if you're called in to see the CEO you won't need to make excuses about being casual.

1. Get Job

YOUR DRESS CODE

Regardless of the dress code employed by your office or industry, over time you will begin to develop your own sense of style and perhaps even some sartorial trademarks. Do you only wear ties with polka dots on them? Are you the kind of man who insists on cowboy boots with a suit? Does everyone notice your cuff links? Whatever your personal dress code is, you must, of course, still look professional. And as you climb the corporate ladder, it will become easier to express your personality through your clothes. After all, who will tell the boss he shouldn't wear pink checked shirts?

LEARNING INDUSTRY DRESS CODES

Just as offices have dress codes, so, too, do industries. And even if your office does not adhere to the industry standard, when you go for an interview or meeting at another office, the best preparation is to research what that company's policy is. Call someone in the human resources department and get a sense of what the guidelines are. In general, industry dress codes have become more relaxed, but a safe rule would be to maintain a high level of dress whenever you are uncertain. Going to a law office? Wear a suit and tie. Meeting people at an advertising agency? Business appropriate would not be inappropriate. Feeling at ease with the way you are dressed will alleviate some of the pressures that you may be feeling about the job itself.

DRESS CODE EXCEPTIONS

Even if you understand your office or industry dress code perfectly, there will still be exceptions to the rules. For instance, you work in a corporate dress code office, but there is an off-site workshop at a local hotel and you have been told you can dress down. The smart move would be to dress business appropriate. Or perhaps you work in a business appropriate office but you are meeting clients for lunch who are business casual. Simple solution: Remove your tie. No matter what the situation is you should always be prepared to adapt your wardrobe and get down to business.

Due Diligence

SHOE TREE
Another smart investment aid—more consistent than your friends' stock tips—shoe trees are cedar molds that fit inside your shoes. They help dry out the sweat of the day, keep the leather from sinking and cracking, and keep your shoes odor-free and new looking.

NO EXCEPTIONS
Want to be sure to create a bad impression in whatever dress code your employer prescribes, or blow your job interview? It's simple: Never polish your shoes, let the heels get worn and the leather cracked. If, however, you would rather make a good impression or land that new job, some preventive maintenance can go a long way.

SHINER
Either go to a pro or spend some time each weekend (15 minutes per pair) polishing your shoes 1. Take a rag that's moist and swirl good wax polish on your shoe in a circular motion. 2. Keep up this motion as the previous shine disappears and is replaced with a deeper shine. 3. Then use another rag and buff to the shine level you prefer. Buy an edge dressing, which is simply a dye to paint the leather edges. Every six months have your shoe repairman check the soles—good for your shoes, good for your career.

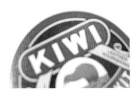

industry guidelines

No industry standard is foolproof—different companies within the same industry often have their own rules—but there are some general guidelines that tend to remain consistent within a particular profession.

Who Wears What to Work

Deciphering Industry Dress Codes

ACADEMIC
Still tweedy after all these years. While suits are not out of the question, most professors tend to wear business appropriate clothes: Jackets and ties, sweaters, turtlenecks, etc.

ACCOUNTING
Those in executive accounting positions tend to dress in corporate attire. But for all other accounting titles—bookkeepers, semisenior accountants, assistants—it's more casual. In smaller accounting firms, corporate casual attire can mean anything from jeans and khakis to a sport jacket. Larger firms, however, often require their paraprofessionals to dress professionally, or business appropriate.

ADVERTISING
Like many creative media, the dress code in advertising tends to be corporate creative. For entry-level positions, that means looking sharp, but not stiff

and too dressed up—a nice pair of pants and a dress shirt should do it. Midlevel employees can take liberties within a corporate casual to business appropriate range, but if they're meeting clients outside the office, they should do their homework and know how the clients dress. Senior executives dress with similar freedom, in everything from Armani to jeans. Clearly, the more conservative the firm—or a particular client—the more conservative the dress code.

ARCHITECTURE
The dress code in architecture is similar to that in advertising: Casual but neat. Business appropriate is always acceptable, but suits are not necessary unless you're meeting clients who are likely to wear them.

FINANCIAL
Banking has eased its dress code in the last decade, but the standard

seems to be regressing. If you don't have to wear a suit, you should at least remain business appropriate.

INTERNET

Ever since the dot-com bubble broke, the dress code for the industry has gotten somewhat more serious. (When your company is worth billions on paper you can wear what you want. When it's no longer worth the paper that paper was printed on, you have to look professional.) Still, business casual to business appropriate is the norm here.

LAW

The law is still very serious business. Corporate dress codes still apply at most white-shoe firms, but you could get away with business appropriate at some smaller firms.

MEDIA

Jobs in the media—television and film production, publishing—generally inspire a creative take on business attire. Anyone who is a figurehead—an editor in chief, a producer—tends to be at the higher end of the style spectrum. But, in general, business casual to business appropriate is the way to dress.

MEDICINE

Aside from the white lab coat, doctors tend to wear a shirt and tie underneath or at least a nice dress shirt. As with everything in medicine, neatness counts.

REAL ESTATE

If you're selling real estate, you want to dress in a manner that your clients can relate to. So, if you're selling high-end homes, dress high-end. Affordable housing? Dress business appropriate.

The key here is making your clients feel, well, at home.

RETAIL

Looking presentable is the goal. Most stores will either want you to wear their clothes or at least represent the clientele. In other words, if you work at a high-end store, you should have a reasonably high standard of dress. After all, if you are recommending a $1,500 suit to someone, you can't be seen in a T-shirt and jeans.

SERVICE INDUSTRY

Service positions—hotel managers, restaurant workers—often require a uniform. Otherwise, the rule of thumb is to wear crisp, well-ironed, and presentable clothes that fall into the business casual or business appropriate range, depending on the position.

FOUR-IN-HAND

Your first goal is to learn how to tie your tie. There are four basic styles, but for your job interview, simple and straightforward is best—the four-in-hand.

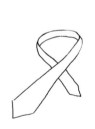 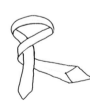 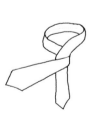 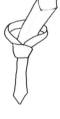 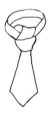 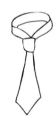

STEP BY STEP

1. Begin with the tie's wide end approximately one foot below the narrow end. Cross it over the narrow end and bring it back underneath.

2. Cross the wide end over again and bring it up through the loop.

3. Holding the front of the knot loosely with the thumb and index finger, take the wide end through the loop in front.

4. Tighten the knot slowly, holding the narrow end and sliding the knot to the collar.

Dressing for Your Goals
—Throughout Your Career

How you dress at a certain point in your career is often based on what level you have attained or hope to attain. Are your clothes ready to climb the ladder of success?

GET A JOB

Whether you are just out of college, between engagements, or looking to get back to work after a layoff of many years, getting a job is your mission. And every detail matters.

The main goal for you is to dress the part and let your potential employer know that you seem competent and would fit in. Research the company and determine how its employees dress. Then outfit your-self accordingly so that your first impression is a good one. (Of course, if you have to alter who you are dramatically just to get a job, perhaps that job isn't right for you after all.) When you step through the door for that initial interview, let them think you already work there.

SUCCEED IN A JOB

Once you're in the door, the object is to stay there. To do that, you need a wardrobe that works overtime right alongside you. It must be filled with versatile clothes that you can wear in every foreseeable situation—and even a few you never saw coming. Once again, though, looking the part will only get you so far. You have to back up your style with substance.

"The ideal look, as you claw your way to the lower middle rung, is that of a hip funeral director…
To the delight of your boss, your sartorial restraint will signify a comforting subservience."

SIMON DOONAN
Author, writer for *The New York Observer*

GET A BETTER JOB

In order to get ahead, you have to dress for the job you want to have, not the job you were hired to do. Reassess yourself. Do you look like the kind of man who can be an authority figure? Do your clothes command respect? Or are you still dressing like someone's slacker assistant?

Now that you've proved yourself for a while, you feel you're entitled to some more money, a bigger office, and greater responsibilities. If your superiors see that you look worthy of a better job it will likely influence them to give you that opportunity.

DRESSING SMART—THROUGHOUT YOUR CAREERS

No job lasts forever. Most career paths are long and winding. As you change jobs, careers, cities, and perhaps even worldviews, reassess your wardrobe and what your goals are. Are you still dressing for your last career? Do your suits look as though they belong in a time capsule? Has your body changed dramatically, but no one notified your clothes? Along the way, every few years, reflect on where you have been and where you are going. Then take a look at your closet and determine if your clothes should come along for the ride.

1. Get Job

Dress Smart
—The Packaging of You

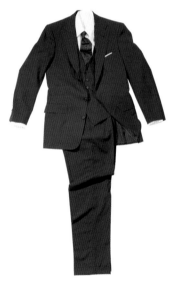

YOUR PERSONAL BRAND
As David McNally and Karl Speak stated so well in *Be Your Own Brand*, "A brand reflects a perception or emotion maintained in somebody else's mind… It doesn't matter nearly as much as you think. It matters a whole lot what other people think."

YOU ARE THE BRAND

With corporations spending millions on establishing brands, redefining brands, and expanding brands, it should come as little surprise that you, too, have a brand: Yourself. And how you package that brand will be integral to the path of your career. By understanding that your identity can be defined by the way you dress and by deciding what clear message you are going to send out, you are defining your image and not allowing others to shape it for you. This is the first important step to taking control of your career.

CLOTHES AS BRAND ATTRIBUTES

Tom Wolfe always wears a white suit. Johnny Cash is the Man in Black. George Will favors bow ties. Pat Riley lives in Armani suits. Men such as these define themselves by what they wear. Their trademark styles immediately telegraph who they are and what they stand for. (Wolfe: "I'm a dandy and a latter-day Mark Twain." Cash: "I've got a dark side." Will: "I'm a conservative brainiac." Riley: "I've got a winning style.")

Signatures such as these have long been understood by politicians. Consider some past presidents: Bill Clinton sported Donna Karan suits, suggesting that he was the very model of a modern man. Ronald Reagan epitomized the man who wears red power ties. Jimmy Carter chose cozy sweaters to imply that he was a warm and fuzzy president, a man of the people. And John F. Kennedy famously brought about the demise of the men's hat because he refused to wear one.

The same principles apply in business. A boss who rolls up his shirt sleeves at work is telling his staff that he is unafraid of hard work. A young assistant who carries a briefcase is letting everyone know how hard he will work and how organized he is. In the early stages of a career, having a signature look is hardly important. In fact, if one is too stylish it may actually be a distraction for many in the office. Early on, you want to show people that you are competent and reliable. There will be plenty of time to amass that Hermès tie collection.

KNOW YOUR AUDIENCE

What may be appropriate in your office may not be ideal for the world at large. Simply following a dress code blindly, without taking your audience into account, can be perilous. For instance, a black suit, which is perfectly acceptable attire in New York City, may seem off-putting and too edgy for those in the South. Likewise, a white-collar manager who works mainly in the office might seem out of place if he dressed in a suit and tie to meet the branch office in the Midwest. The message you are delivering may be loud and clear, but you may be delivering it to deaf ears.

THE CONVERSATION YOU NEVER HEAR

Like ancient Greek poetry, an office dress code is rarely written down. When you are hired, you are unlikely to be told how to dress for your first day on the job, and this may leave you flummoxed. So what can you do? Simple: Look around you and ask. When you went on inter-views, what were the people who hired you wearing? What were the people who work for them wearing? Pay attention and follow suit. If that fails and you are still unsure, ask before you begin. It will only reflect well on you—one more example of how conscientious you are.

Similarly, if you have already been working somewhere and you are inappropriately dressed, you may not hear it until it is too late. Don't show an employer a weakness such as poor dressing. It's too easy a mistake to correct to let it put a detour on your career path. So pay attention to your peers. Who knows, the dress code may be changing right before your eyes and you were busy waiting for the memo.

1. Get Job

Dress Better, Spend Less: Wardrobe Economics

DRESSING FOR THE JOB INTERVIEW

You spent years getting the education, weeks setting up the appointments, and days polishing the résumé, so don't let a few minutes of bad clothes or poor grooming undermine all that. This is your first, and perhaps only, encounter with a potential employer, and you need to make the most of it.

Think of a job interview as a blind date, albeit a professional one. You and your interviewer have a finite amount of time to figure out if you have similar interests, compatible work ethics and skill sets, and whether you are comfortable enough with one another to spend eight hours a day together. And, just as on a blind date, you want to make the best first impression. Appearance counts. It's not that you have to be attractive to an interviewer, but you do have to appear professional and highly competent—because if you don't, the next guy will.

INVEST IN YOURSELF

Preparing for a career comes with start-up costs, but there will be a return on investment—a salary. While it may hurt the bottom line at first to buy a suit, shirts, ties, and a nice pair of shoes, you have to trust in your ability to get a job and understand that this will be a relatively low-risk investment. The right suit, paired with a good shirt and tie, will provide you with enough confidence to walk into any interviewer's office. It's a confidence that speaks not only to your skills as a potential employee, but also provides you with peace of mind; while interviewing, you shouldn't be thinking about what you're wearing.

DOLLARS AND GOOD SENSE

Tempting as it may be to go out and purchase an expensive first suit, it would be very unwise. Looking good has nothing to do with how much money you spend, and at this point in your life, why blow your budget on a $1,500 suit, when one for $250 will suffice? You need to determine what your greatest needs are and then understand where to put the most money and where not to.

SHOP SMART. QUALITY = VALUE

If splurging on an Armani suit isn't the answer right now, what is? Quality. Whether it's a handsome suit or a good pair of shoes, it is more important to buy items of quality rather than name-brand designs. To understand how quality can make a difference, go to a department store and try on some high-end suits—notice how they are constructed, how the fabric feels to the hand. Then, head over to the cheaper racks and look for suits that resemble (in fit and fabric) the pricey versions you just tried on.

WARDROBE ECONOMICS

To dress well without spending a fortune requires foresight. If you know what you are willing to spend the most on, and roughly how high you can afford to go, you will be a much smarter shopper. One of the most basic rules when starting out is to stick with the classics: Blue suits, white shirts, simple black lace-up shoes. These items can last you for years and will never go out of style.

The majority of your investment should go to that first suit. After all, it is the armor that will protect you as you head off to interview, and you need to be flawless. A single-breasted navy suit in medium-weight wool is the way to go. You can wear it all year, and it won't go out of style before your third promotion.

Think about the elements that will go best with it: Shirts, ties, shoes. And again, remember that you don't need to spend a lot to get good quality: A $25 tie can look just as sharp as a $150 tie.

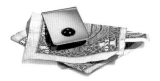

REALITY CHECK
Whether you are graduating from school with a small national debt in student loans or were recently laid off, the idea of spending money on clothes may appear laughable. Deal with it; if you don't have the vision and courage to bet on yourself then what's the point? It always hurts to win but so does losing. Pay attention, read carefully, make a list and stick to it. You are buying your uniform for your first job, a new job, a new start—what could be money better spent?

1. Get Job

Get the Job—No Excuses

BE PREPARED
Employers say that candidates who manage to land interviews are increasingly unprepared—sometimes woefully so—for the interviewing process. "Many can't provide details to probing questions," said Paige Soltano, senior partner for Bozell New York, an advertising agency. "If they tell you they completed a successful project at their old job, and you ask them why it was successful, they aren't able to give you any details."
New York Times
8/8/01

You never get a second chance to make a first impression, and nothing is more professional looking than a suit with a shirt and tie. It's strong, authoritative, and shows that you're serious about what you do for a living. Is it enough to get you the job? Maybe not, but the proper attire will send the right message: You're ready for business.

GIVING GOOD INTERVIEW
There are five elements to consider when preparing for an interview. Each one will get you closer to your ultimate goal.

1. **Be confident.** Perhaps no attribute is more important for an interviewee than confidence. It signals to the interviewer that you can handle responsibility, authority, pressure, and, above all, that you can deliver. And even if you don't actually have confidence, there are some smart ways to fake it. Look the other person in the eyes when you firmly shake hands. Sit up tall. Be articulate. But mostly, just be yourself.

2. **Be prepared.** Anyone who's ever been a Boy Scout understands the importance of this credo. If you want to know where the confidence comes from, it's right here—so know your stuff. Read up on the company and read up on yourself (which means, know your own résumé). Anticipate the questions you might be asked. Look into whether you and your interviewer have any people or hobbies in common—anything to give you an edge.

3. **Be knowledgeable.** By researching the industry and the company itself you will have intelligent questions ready if you're asked. After all, you're not the only one who is being interviewed here. You're just the one without a job.
4. **Be enthusiastic.** What you may lack in experience, you can certainly make up for with enthusiasm. Companies constantly need new blood, and that's what you provide, so don't be anemic. Your enthusiasm should be infectious.
5. **Be the man.** Once you have the four other elements, you can focus on the outward presentation: Your clothes, your hair, your delivery. When you've got that nailed down, the job will be yours to lose.

HERE COMES THE GROOMING

Being the best-dressed man in the room won't mean a thing if your hair looks dirty, you haven't shaved, and your nails could earn you a spot in the *Guinness Book of World Records*. Grooming counts. Make sure your hair looks neat (which is not to be confused with short; if you wear your hair long, that's fine, just make sure it's trimmed and shampooed regularly). As for facial hair, clean-shaven is always the safest way to go, but if you do wear a mustache or beard, keep it neatly trimmed—leave the scraggly facial hair to the guys in ZZ Top. Nails, meanwhile, should be clipped at least once a month. Get yourself a nail trimmer and wash your hands regularly to get the dirt out. Finally, if you're the kind of man you wears cologne, make sure that only those people who come in close contact with your neck know you wear it. The whole office didn't agree to wear your scent.

THE DRESS REHEARSAL

A day or so before your interview, put your outfit on. Move around in it. Get used to sitting down in your suit or crossing your legs, anything that might be awkward. Does the jacket fit like you thought it would? Are the pants wrinkled? The idea is to be as comfortable as possible in these clothes, so you don't get distracted.

Next, make a list of all the things you want to bring to the interview (résumés, pens, notepad), and have some questions you might have for your interviewer ready to go. All of this preparation will only fuel your confidence, and assuming you present your best self, then… well…

1. Get Job

ENTITLEMENT
All right, let's deal with the simple gold hoop, the tasteful stud, a simple drop pendant, the feathered hand-carved wooden fetish original ear art picked up in Fiji—is it acceptable and do you wear it or not? It's your call, just like goatees, beards, dreads, necklaces, and bracelets. Your freedom to wear what you choose is not in question but your right to have a particular job is in the eye of the beholder who is offering the job. If it's important to you to express your individuality, then the employer who finds these elements uncomfortable will probably not hire you. If the opportunity the job offers is worth some self-adjustment, well, perhaps you can sacrifice some style points.

CONGRATULATIONS: THE SECOND INTERVIEW

Okay, so you made a nice impression, but now what do you wear the second time around? Clearly you need a variation on a theme here, so go for a different shirt-and-tie combination with the same suit. If you wore a white shirt on the first interview, try blue for the second. Remember, the jacket is just the frame, the shirt and tie are the picture.

ENOUGH ALREADY. THE THIRD CALLBACK

Well, clearly it's looking good. If you get asked back again, it's almost always a sure sign that the job is yours. Usually the third meeting is with the boss himself, so be at the top of your game. Go back to the white shirt with your blue suit and try a different tie. Your suit's been busy lately so make sure it's pressed. The last thing you want to do is appear wrinkled in front of the boss.

SPECIAL CIRCUMSTANCES: BREAKFAST, LUNCH, DINNER, ETC.

If one of your interviews is scheduled for a meal, don't lose your lunch over it. Yes, table manners will come into play, but the same rules apply: Dress just as you would for an office meeting. And whatever you do, don't order a drink to relax yourself. Especially at breakfast.

shop smart

The first items you purchase for your career will make up the interview wardrobe. In the following field guide, we will break down the various elements that go into this wardrobe and explain how to get the most impact with the least amount of money.

An interview suit needs to be bulletproof: Something that looks perfect on you and makes you feel confident and secure about the person who fills it out. When matched with a simple shirt-and-tie combination, the outfit should make you look like you've worked at the company for years.

And, with any luck, you will.

How to Buy an Interview Suit

COLOR
Navy. It's sophisticated enough to wear anywhere, any time, any season. And every other color—gray, brown, red, green, even black—mixes with it easily and effortlessly.

JACKET CUT
Timeless style: Single-breasted, two-button with medium lapels. Center vent or no vent, your call. The hem of the jacket should fall roughly where your fist ends when your arms hang down. The sleeves should allow for a 1/2" of shirt cuff to show. Shoulders should be padded to make you look formidable—but not so much that you're ready for the NFL.
Pants: There are only two decisions: Flat front or pleated? Each is perfectly appropriate in the workplace, but flat front is more slimming. The other choice is cuffs or no cuffs. There is no choice. Get your suit trousers cuffed:

1 1/2". This will give the pants the proper break at the instep.
Fabric: Wool is your only selection here, and worsted is best. It's heavy enough to wear in colder weather and light enough for summer. This allows your suit to be as versatile as possible.

FIT
Get the suit tailored properly, either in the store or by your local tailor. Before you see the tailor, though, walk around a bit, then stand in front of a three-way mirror and ask yourself a few questions: Can you button the jacket? Can you breathe when it's buttoned? Can you move your arms comfortably? Does it bulge in the back? Can you sit in it? Do the pants have enough room in the waist? Too much? Is the seat too tight? Did you look at the price tag? When you've satisfied these criteria, you're ready to buy your first suit.

Interview Wardrobe

What you wear on an interview doesn't have to dazzle the person you're meeting—in fact, it's probably best if he or she hardly even notices what you're wearing. So what kind of impression are you making if no one can even remember what you had on? The appropriate one. In a suit with a simple shirt-and-tie combination you will be dressed smartly for an interview. Now you have to act it.

"At one time, the most qualified person got the job. Today, in a situation where three people with equal qualifications are interviewed for a job, the one with the best communication skills gets it."

ROGER AILES
You Are the Message

WHAT DO YOUR CLOTHES SAY TO THE INTERVIEWER?

SHIRT
Sensible
or
Boring?

TIE
Authoritative
or
Fussy?

THREE BUTTONS
Stodgy
or
Trendy?

BELT BUCKLE
Pulled together
or
Pretentious?

PANT CUFFS
Fastidious
or
Foppish?

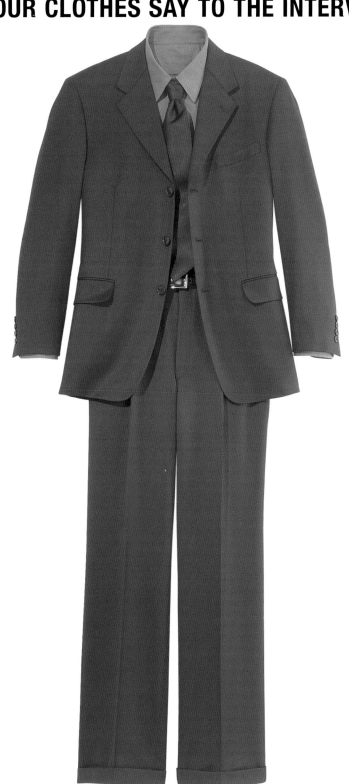

Suit Jacket

Since a suit is essentially the most expensive investment you will be making toward a new job, it pays to get your money's worth. A navy suit will work harder than the other suits in the closet because the jacket can double as a blue blazer, giving you a greater return on your investment.

ALIGNMENT
If the buttons on the jacket don't align when closed, it may not fit properly.

POCKETS
The best way to ensure that the suit pockets don't bulge out? Don't open them.

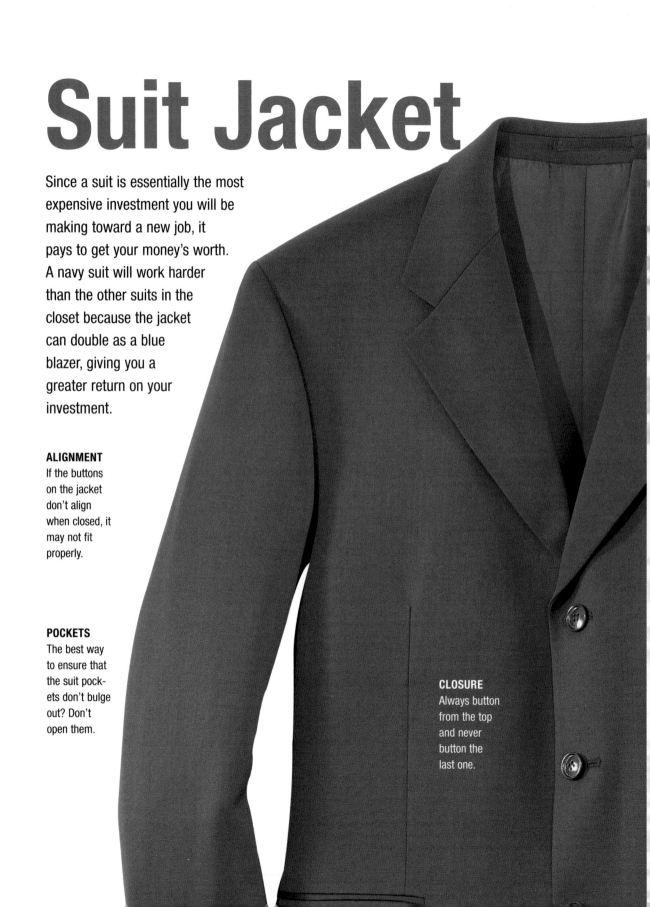

CLOSURE
Always button from the top and never button the last one.

Suit Pants

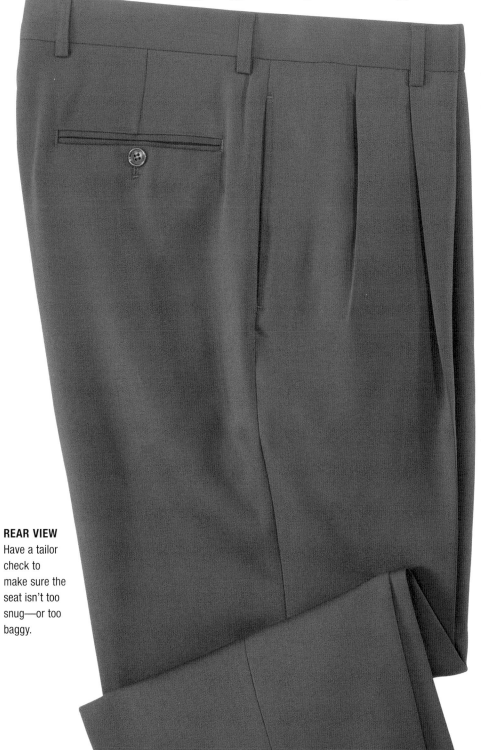

WAIST
Even if you want to wear suspenders, always get a suit with belt loops.

PLEATS VS. FLAT
Pleated pants may be better suited for larger men, but flat-front trousers will be more slimming.

REAR VIEW
Have a tailor check to make sure the seat isn't too snug—or too baggy.

Shirts

As important as wearing the right suit is to a man, a shirt and tie allow him to express his individuality. Select a shirt that sends the best message about who you are.

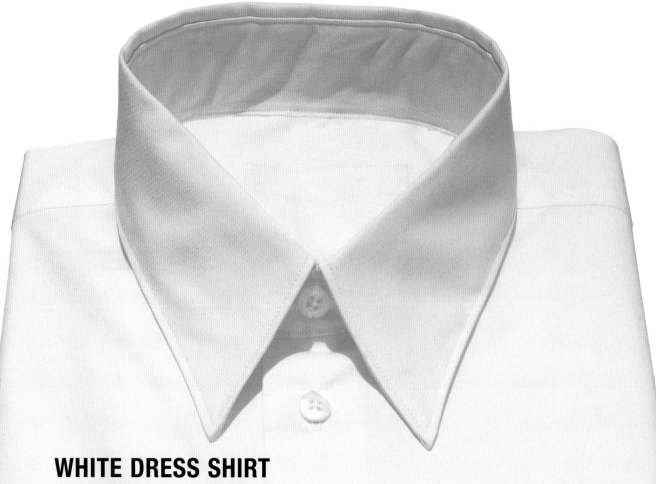

WHITE DRESS SHIRT

KEY POINTS: Straight collar of medium length. Button cuffs. Broadcloth.

There is no occasion for which a white shirt is inappropriate. It goes with everything from a sport jacket to khakis to jeans, and when paired with a suit it sends just the right message: Neat and efficient. A white shirt with this collar works with any face shape and any coloring, but it will all be in vain if it isn't cleaned and pressed properly.

BLUE DRESS SHIRT

KEY POINTS: Straight collar of medium length. Button cuffs. Made of end-on-end cotton, which faintly shows the cross-stitch weave.

Like a white shirt, blue is an all-purpose choice. And in some ways it may be better. Whereas white may reveal a certain conformity, a blue dress shirt signals that you are your own man. Once again, keep it clean and pressed, and wear a white T-shirt underneath to keep it dry.

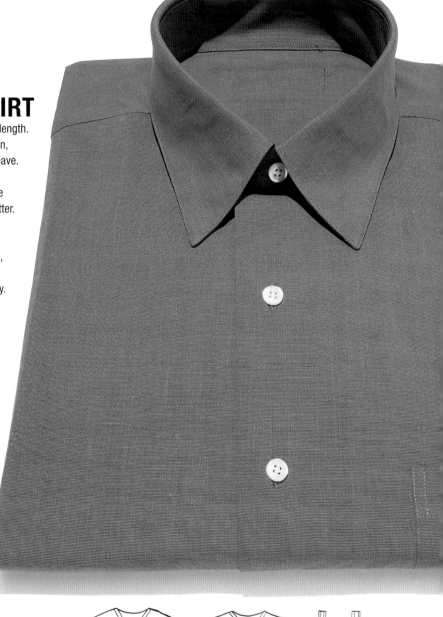

NEVER LET 'EM SEE YOU SWEAT

Interviewing can be a stressful-enough process without having to worry about perspiration. The best defense against it? A white cotton undershirt. Although perhaps counterintuitive because it requires putting on another layer, a white crew neck or V-neck T-shirt will keep dress shirts looking drier and make white shirts even brighter.

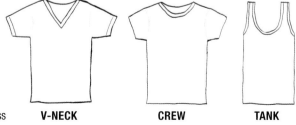

V-NECK   **CREW**   **TANK**

Ties

Perhaps nothing signals a man's individuality more than a tie. In theory, you could wear the same suit and shirt every day—don't— but by changing ties, it would all look new. And yet, men often get tied up in knots trying to decide what to buy.

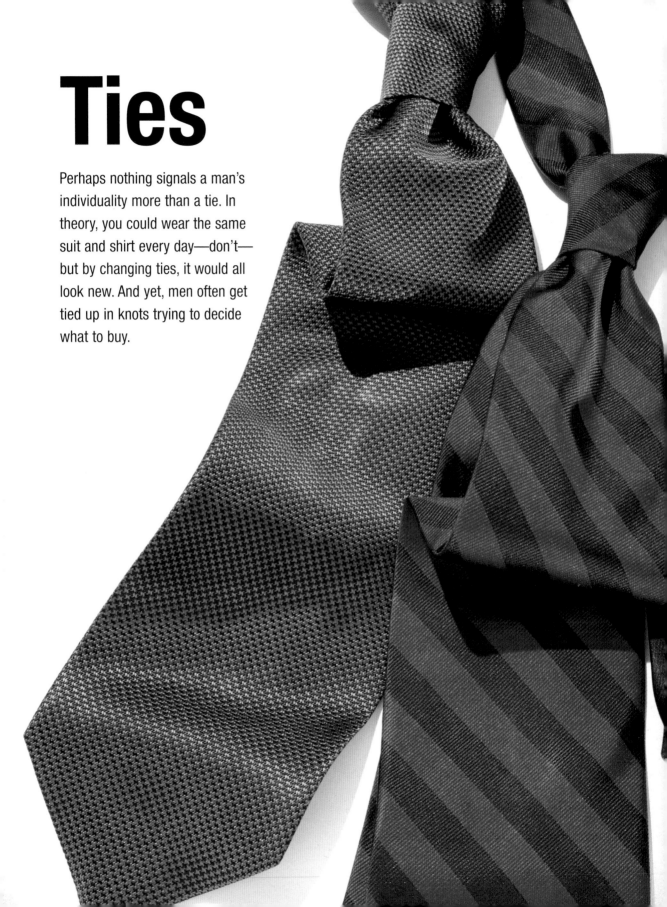

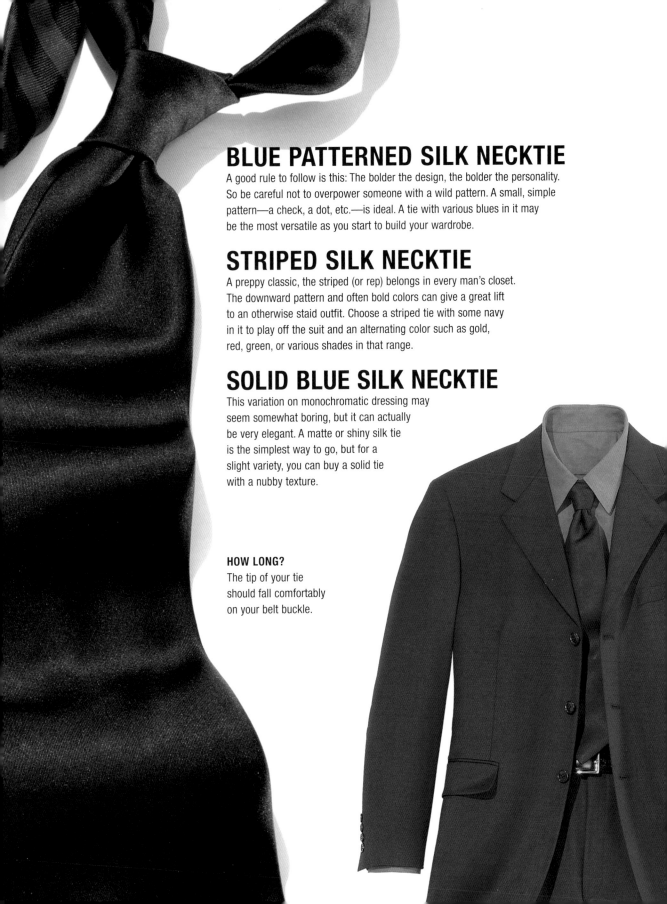

BLUE PATTERNED SILK NECKTIE

A good rule to follow is this: The bolder the design, the bolder the personality. So be careful not to overpower someone with a wild pattern. A small, simple pattern—a check, a dot, etc.—is ideal. A tie with various blues in it may be the most versatile as you start to build your wardrobe.

STRIPED SILK NECKTIE

A preppy classic, the striped (or rep) belongs in every man's closet. The downward pattern and often bold colors can give a great lift to an otherwise staid outfit. Choose a striped tie with some navy in it to play off the suit and an alternating color such as gold, red, green, or various shades in that range.

SOLID BLUE SILK NECKTIE

This variation on monochromatic dressing may seem somewhat boring, but it can actually be very elegant. A matte or shiny silk tie is the simplest way to go, but for a slight variety, you can buy a solid tie with a nubby texture.

HOW LONG?
The tip of your tie should fall comfortably on your belt buckle.

Shoes

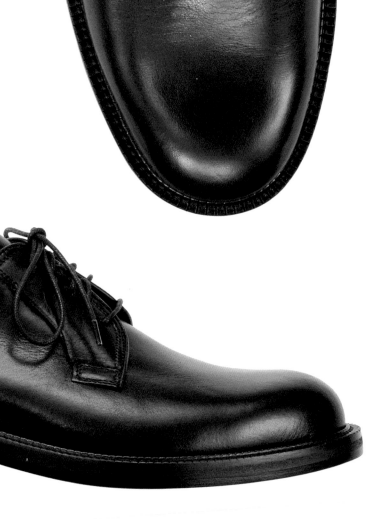

OXFORD

It may be simple—plain black leather with three to six sets of eyelets—but the oxford is the dressiest option for business. Just about the only statement you can make with an oxford is in the toe. Whether it's narrow and traditional (the shoe your father would select) or rounder, with a thicker sole and slightly more hip, keep the plain-toe oxford polished and replace the heels as they wear down. And buy a set of shoe trees.

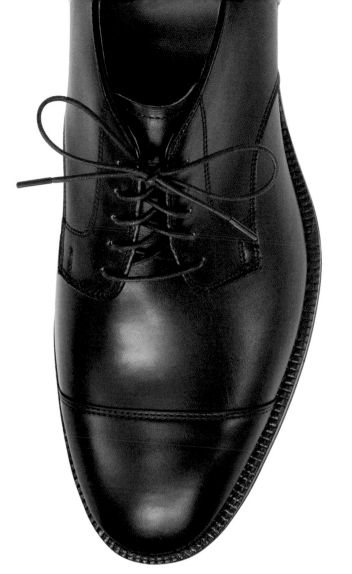

The sole of a man often reveals his soul. Shoes that are well polished, with heels that are not worn down and laces that aren't frayed, are the mark of a man who is responsible and cares about details. Here's how to set off on the right foot.

CAP-TOE OXFORD

A basic variation on the oxford shoe, the cap-toe has a horizontal stitch going across its tip. It's a little more polished than its plain cousin. Unlike the plain oxford, the cap-toe usually comes with a narrow toe.

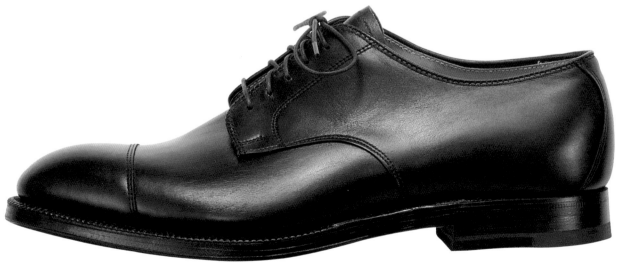

Essentials

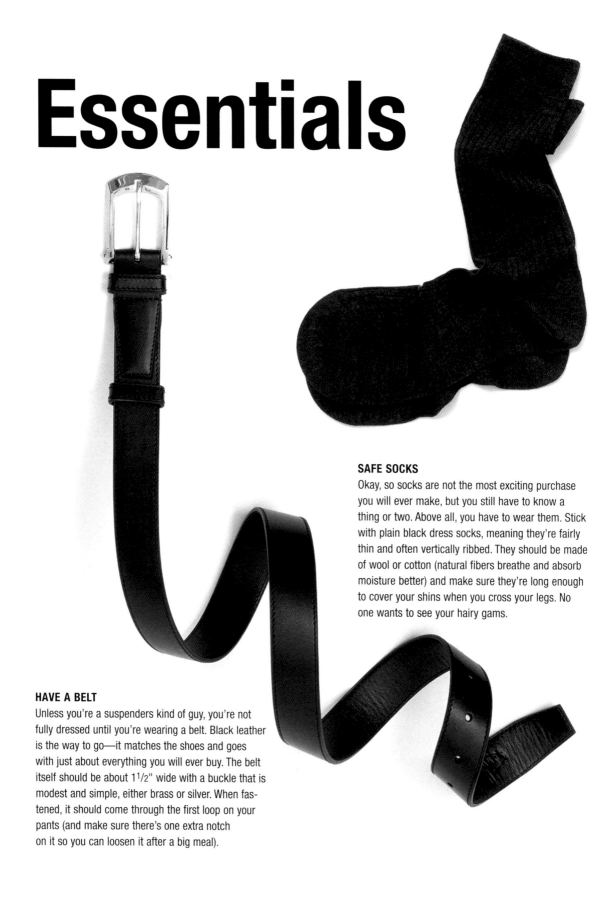

SAFE SOCKS

Okay, so socks are not the most exciting purchase you will ever make, but you still have to know a thing or two. Above all, you have to wear them. Stick with plain black dress socks, meaning they're fairly thin and often vertically ribbed. They should be made of wool or cotton (natural fibers breathe and absorb moisture better) and make sure they're long enough to cover your shins when you cross your legs. No one wants to see your hairy gams.

HAVE A BELT

Unless you're a suspenders kind of guy, you're not fully dressed until you're wearing a belt. Black leather is the way to go—it matches the shoes and goes with just about everything you will ever buy. The belt itself should be about 1^1/$_2$" wide with a buckle that is modest and simple, either brass or silver. When fastened, it should come through the first loop on your pants (and make sure there's one extra notch on it so you can loosen it after a big meal).

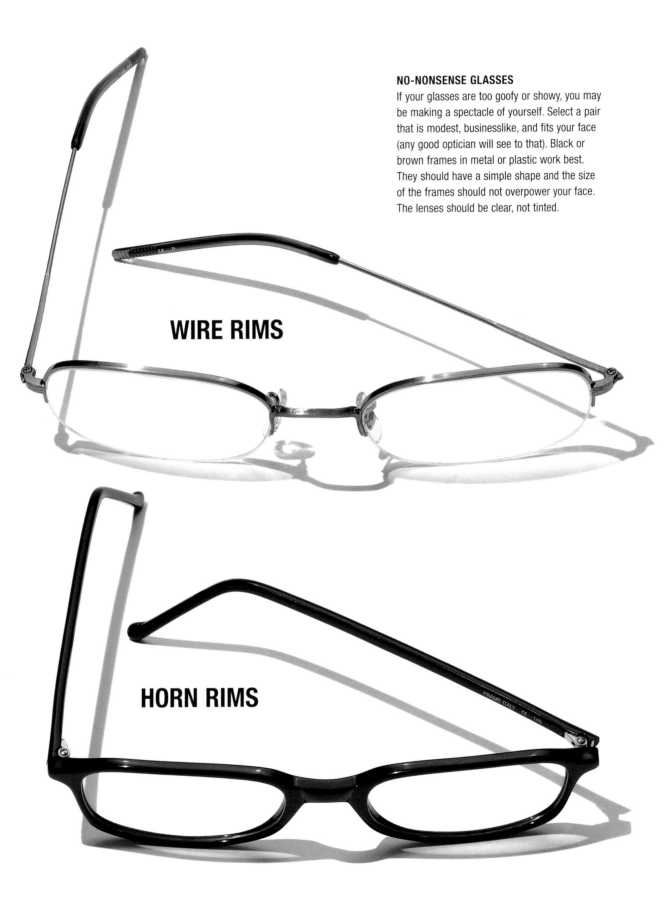

NO-NONSENSE GLASSES
If your glasses are too goofy or showy, you may be making a spectacle of yourself. Select a pair that is modest, businesslike, and fits your face (any good optician will see to that). Black or brown frames in metal or plastic work best. They should have a simple shape and the size of the frames should not overpower your face. The lenses should be clear, not tinted.

WIRE RIMS

HORN RIMS

Résumé/Portfolio

One last detail before you walk into that interview: Carry a black leather agenda or planner. It can hold extra résumés, and you can write down any information you might need later. Above all, it says that you are organized.

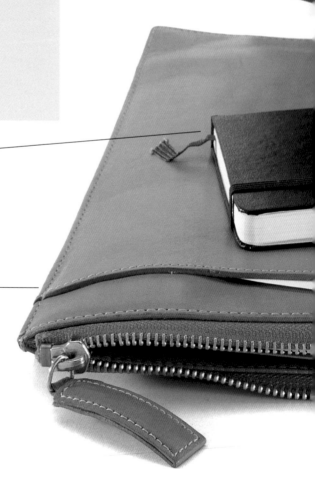

INTERVIEW CHECKLIST

Better safe than sorry when heading out to an interview. Here are some last-minute items to consider:

1. Two pens (in case one runs out)
2. Wallet or money clip
3. Interview contact's name, address, and phone number
4. Extra résumés
5. Date book or PDA (to schedule future appointments)
6. Cell phone (turn it off before the interview)
7. Breath mints

AGENDA
Got a follow-up interview? Write it down in your agenda. It will make you look efficient. And if an agenda is too old-fashioned for you, try a PDA.

LEATHER PORTFOLIO
More sophisticated than the plastic box, the leather portfolio can also double as your first briefcase.

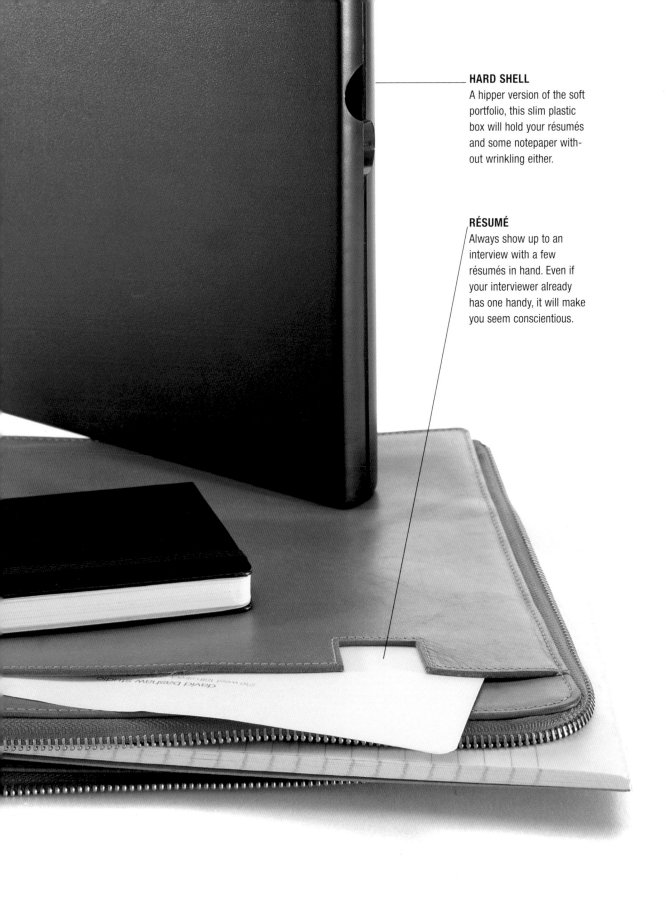

HARD SHELL
A hipper version of the soft portfolio, this slim plastic box will hold your résumés and some notepaper without wrinkling either.

RÉSUMÉ
Always show up to an interview with a few résumés in hand. Even if your interviewer already has one handy, it will make you seem conscientious.

Watch

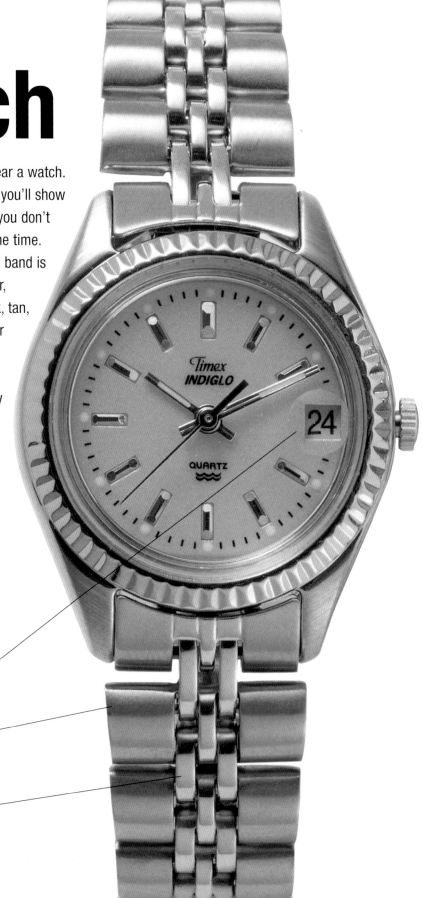

Every working man should wear a watch. It doesn't cost that much and you'll show up early for your interview. If you don't have the right watch, now's the time. Either a leather strap or metal band is appropriate for work. If leather, select a smooth band in black, tan, or brown. With metal, consider stainless steel or gold (or a combination of the two), but don't wear anything too flashy or sporty. A simple round or rectangular face is ideal. Save the digital for the gym.

Easy to read, but not digital, which is too sporty.

Round or rectangular face are equally appropriate.

A versatile, stainless steel and gold combination matches both gold and silver jewelry.

Asset: Date indicator.

Integral bracelet.

Light-colored background face.

Link, not expansion, band.

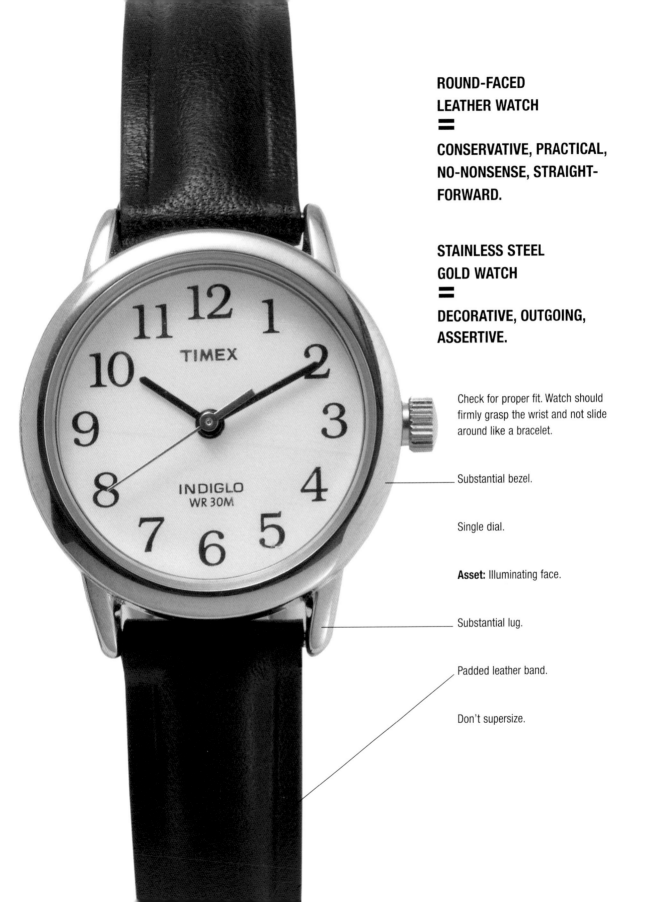

ROUND-FACED LEATHER WATCH
=
CONSERVATIVE, PRACTICAL, NO-NONSENSE, STRAIGHT-FORWARD.

STAINLESS STEEL GOLD WATCH
=
DECORATIVE, OUTGOING, ASSERTIVE.

Check for proper fit. Watch should firmly grasp the wrist and not slide around like a bracelet.

Substantial bezel.

Single dial.

Asset: Illuminating face.

Substantial lug.

Padded leather band.

Don't supersize.

CLOSET 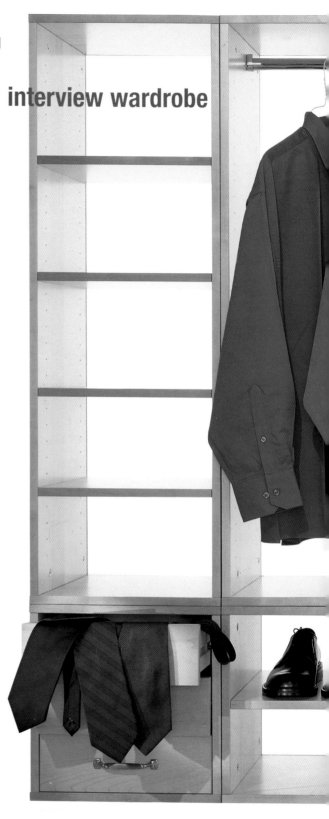 interview wardrobe

Your closet will be mostly full of nonwork clothes at this point in your career, which means that organizing what you wear to the office will be relatively simple. Here is a list of the minimum you should have in your work wardrobe as well as the accessories you will need to maintain your clothes properly:

INTERVIEW WARDROBE

1 suit
3 shirts
3 ties
1 pair of shoes

1 watch
1 portfolio
socks/underwear

CLOSET TOOLS

- Full-length mirror
- Good lighting
- Solid hangers (to help maintain the shape of your clothes)

- Shoe trees
- Lint remover
- Iron/ironing board
- Steamer

CLOTHES CHECK

- Avoid dry-cleaning your clothes too often as it can be hard on fabrics. (Worn often—dry-clean twice a month; worn weekly—once a month; worn occasionally—once a season.)
- Instead of dry-cleaning wrinkled suits, try steaming them (either with a steamer or by hanging them in the bathroom while you take a hot shower).
- Hang up your suit or sport jacket every night, and place shoe trees in your shoes when you take them off.
- Remove clothes from dry-cleaning bags when you get them home. They tend to yellow whites and hold in moisture.

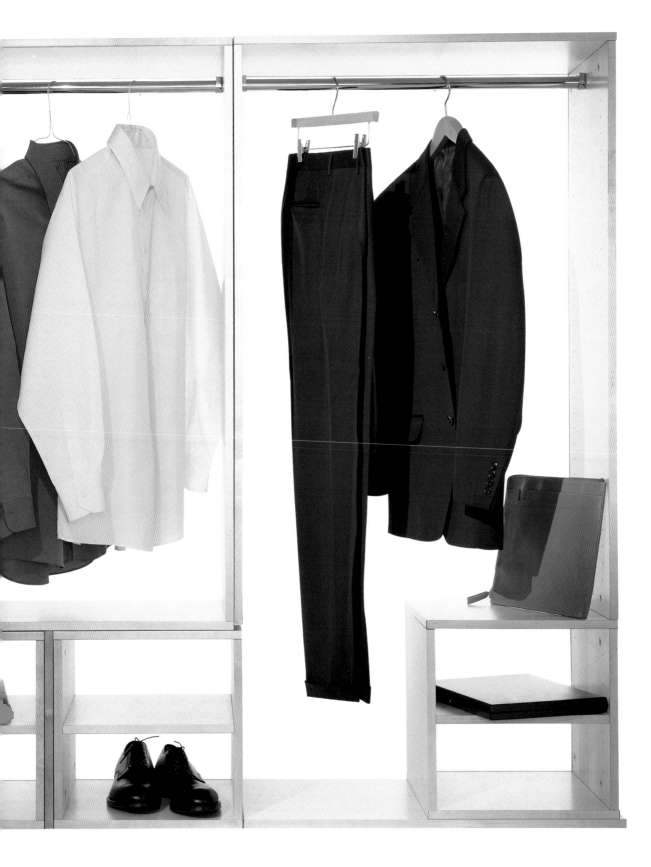

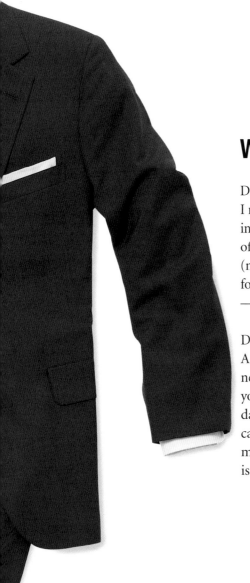

WHAT SUITS YOU?

Dear jeff and Kim,
I recently landed a management position similar to my last job, but in my previous job I wore a suit only when clients came to the office. In my new job the only casual days are Fridays. My two suits (navy and tan) aren't going to cut it but I can't afford to buy one for every day. Is there a simple answer or do I just buy lots of ties?
—Closet Challenged

Dear Closet Challenged,
A navy and gray suit will take you far, so make the gray suit your next purchase. Spend a little more on this suit and it will become your bulletproof outfit. Also, add a blazer or sport coat in a small dark pattern to look pulled together on casual Fridays. Spend carefully on some good cotton shirts and silk ties and you can make it seem as if your wardrobe is endless. Remember, the suit is just the frame, the shirt and tie are the picture.

—jeff and Kim

Succeed 2 in Job

Work Wardrobe

Stuff comes out of work. Paychecks, promotions, and at one time, even security. But that has disappeared. The only security left is your ability to do well, take care of yourself, and present a clear, distinct message of your ability and worth. No matter your skill set, it is essential that you not worry about the impression you are making. Your clothes should be taking care of the silent dialogue that happens whether you're walking down a hallway in your office, seeing a customer, or sitting in a meeting. In this section, options are presented for you to build a wardrobe that will save you money and send an unmistakable message of your value and competence (if you're not competent and don't have value—your clothes won't help).

2. Succeed in Job

Dress Like You Mean Business

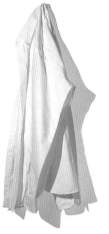

**THANK YOU,
JOHN MOLLOY**
Men who wore white shirts
were thought to be more
competent and honest...
Dress for Success, 1976
(Men in white shirts) are
more intelligent, honest,
successful and powerful
than men wearing any
other color.
Dress for Success, 1988

WELCOME ABOARD

How you dress in an interview is one thing, but what you wear to work every day once you have the position is quite another and far more complicated. The former involves looking the part and instantly communicating to your potential employers that you belong. But once you have the job, it is important to maintain appearances and standards. Obviously, your performance at work will not be judged based on how you look, but in other important ways dressing smart is essential for succeeding in the workplace.

MEN OF RESPECT

Dressing appropriately in the office is a sign of respect. It tells your coworkers and superiors that you are ready for business every single day. And the truth is, it does not take that much effort to dress properly for the office. In fact, that's the point: If you can't take the time to care about your appearance, then you are telling everyone that perhaps you aren't taking proper care of your professional responsibilities, either.

This is the true lesson behind dressing smart in the office: You are ultimately showing respect for yourself. And if you do that, others will as well.

Your Work Wardrobe
—Ensuring Image Control

> "If I can be one step ahead because of the clothes I wear, then it's worth it."
>
> **CRAIG POGSON**
> Maître d' at Orsay

Every industry has different standards, every company within an industry has different standards, and often there are divisions within the same company that have different standards than other divisions. That said, there are some basic principles to follow when dressing for work, and they will always apply:

1. **Be appropriate**. An office or industry is like a club. Look like you're a member, not a guest.
2. **Be professional.** Whether your code is corporate or casual, the clothes you wear should always reflect your seriousness about business. This will give you a quiet confidence that you can handle any task.
3. **Be comfortable.** You cannot dress like someone you're not. If you feel comfortable only in blue suits, then wear them. Dress for your personality and body type. But remember, comfortable does not mean sloppy.
4. **Be strategic.** Clothes can set you apart. Ask yourself what your goals are and then dress accordingly. Are you looking for a promotion? Try wearing bolder ties so you stand out more. Is your profile too high and you just want to be part of the team? Start dressing more like the other players. Do you want the boss to notice you more? Pay attention to how he dresses, mimic him (within your budget, of course), and let him compliment you on your good taste.

2. Succeed in Job

BEING APPROPRIATE: ONE LESS THING TO WORRY ABOUT

Fourteen voice-mail messages after lunch. Thirty-two e-mails to return. A PowerPoint presentation coming up in three weeks. There are enough pressures in the office these days without having to worry about what you wear every day. If you can maximize your wardrobe's potential and learn the principles of smart dressing, you will remove (or at least reduce) a potential source of professional anxiety. Even the simple task of planning an outfit the night before an important meeting or lunch can ease your mind so that you walk in fully prepared.

WORK EMERGENCY KIT: DESK

We all grew up with "be prepared" as a male mantra. In adolescence we carried our "prepared" in our wallets and nowadays the less exciting jumper cables in the car. Being prepared is also good at work, especially since you never want to be unprepared for fate. So if you get a chance to shine be sure your shoes do, too. Always keep the following quick saves in your desk drawer.

❏ Clean white shirt pressed and wrapped from the cleaners

❏ A solid or tonal dark tie

❏ Deodorant

❏ Toothbrush and toothpaste

❏ A comb

❏ Disposable quick wipe shoe buffer

❏ Spare set of shoelaces

❏ Spare set of collar stays

❏ Sewing kit from a hotel or travel kit

❏ Nail clippers

❏ Eye drops

❏ Disposable razor and small travel shave foam

Didn't Get the Memo

"It is awfully important to know what is and what is not your business."

GERTRUDE STEIN

THE TIMES ARE CHANGING—ARE YOU?

In the mid-90s, as the economy grew exponentially, many established companies embraced the notion of casual Fridays and some firms even abolished dress codes altogether. When you're making that much money, who really cares what your employees are wearing to work?

But as the economy started to turn, it was no longer acceptable to be so laid-back about one's appearance. And when people began to lose their jobs, looking serious about work became a priority again. Consequently, people are showing up early, working late, and finding safety behind a jacket and tie. Or didn't you get that memo?

WHO GOT THE MEMO? LOOK AROUND

Has the office dress code changed in the last few months? Have you even noticed? Look around. Has your boss stopped wearing khakis to work? Has a bohemian colleague shaved and cut his hair shorter? Are you the only one wearing jeans?

Chances are, your colleagues have been dressing up again for work, and if you haven't been, now is the time to dress smarter.

A Chic Simple Review

> "I'm a self-made man, but I think if I had to do it over again, I'd call in someone else."
>
> **ROLAND YOUNG**
> Actor

Now that you've been on the job for a while, it may be time to evaluate your career and your wardrobe: Are they giving you what you want? Or need?

ASSESS: ARE YOU WHERE YOU WANT TO BE?

Is your career going the way you thought it would? Are you doing the kinds of things that challenge you and make you happy? Have you stopped setting your alarm in the morning? If things are going well, where do you want to be five or ten years from now—and what will it take to get there?

Now look at your closet: Is it filled with the kinds of clothes that have supported your goals? Could your closet be holding you back? Do your work clothes draw stares from colleagues? Do they make you sit up straight and work harder?

DEJUNK: WHAT IS HOLDING YOU BACK?

If you're not where you want to be, what is holding you back? Did you set unrealistic goals and expectations for yourself? Are you too hard on yourself? Too easy? Have friends been passing you by? Getting promotions? Taking on greater responsibilities? Is money as important as you thought it was? Is it more important than you care to admit? Is your wardrobe too junior now that you are more senior?

> ## "It's always better to be looked over than over-looked."
>
> **MAE WEST**

RENEW: COMMIT TO THE GOALS YOU'VE MADE

Once you've determined what's holding you back, it's time to figure out what you want to accomplish next—and how to get there. Find a mentor: Someone who can counsel you about your career and shoot straight without offending you. Be proactive about your future: Research other departments in your company or other companies altogether.

Now take a look at your closet. Do you look like the people you admire professionally? Are they dressing with a certain authority that you respond to? Perhaps it's time to look into another clothing investment to take your career to the next level.

BUILDING A CAREER WARDROBE

The reality is, a man could wear the same suit three times a week and no one would notice. A blue suit, if pressed or steamed properly, would look new every day if you paired it with the right shirts and ties, and occasionally threw in a sweater or two. By mixing up what you wear—a striped shirt one day, then blue, then white, then a bold color—you can stretch your limited wardrobe by buying suits of higher quality and being creative with the combinations. Although you may lack in quantity, you can now buy a finer suit that will last longer and follow you up the corporate ladder.

DON'T TAKE FRIDAYS OFF

Even if your office believes in casual Fridays, it doesn't mean you have to. There's no actual rule that says you have to look casual. And if you're looking for a promotion or a raise, why risk looking laid-back on the one day that your boss may take notice of you? Think of yourself like a team looking to make the play-offs—you can't let down in the stretch. So go the extra step to look your best when you want to move up. You never know who's paying attention.

The ROI Wardrobe
—Return on Investment

"It is very
well in
practice,
but it will
never work
in theory."

**FRENCH
MANAGEMENT
SAYING**

INVESTING IN YOUR FUTURE

Beginning a career, like launching a business, comes with start-up costs. Some of these will be obvious (suits cost a fair amount of money) and some will seem hidden (tailoring, dry-cleaning, etc.), but none of them should break you. A plan to spend your money is the key to spending it wisely.

UNDERSTANDING NECESSARY EXPENDITURES

Things to keep in mind when building your wardrobe:

1. You might already own some of the items you need.
2. Choose one or two items to invest in—a suit and a sport jacket—and spend less on the rest.
3. Men are often judged by the shoes and the watch they wear; consider investing in these or at least choose wisely.
4. Easy ways to save: Seasonal sales, sample sales, designer outlets (be careful of irregular items and those with slight imperfections).
5. Go easy spending money on shirts. They wear out, get stained, and the same version can always be purchased again in six months to a year.
6. Choose ties that can work with almost every jacket you own. This will make them stretch further.
7. Ignore trends. Buying the occasional fashionable tie is to be expected, but in general, stick with styles that will never go out of style.

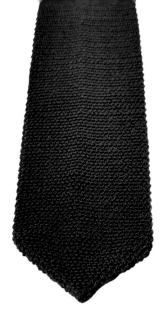

MEET JOE FRIDAY

When contemplating your Friday wardrobe, to tie or not to tie? There's a perfect candidate for the job (hey, just like you)! The black knit tie. It's texture will soften any suit, but will add a bit of polish to a casual shirt or sport coat. It should be tied with a four-in-hand knot to ensure that you don't look like grandpa (which isn't a bad thing—when you *are* his age). The black knit tie is a classic that is welcome in any man's closet. Nice to meet ya', Joe.

SO WHERE DO I BUDGET MY MONEY?

$	**SHIRTS, TIES, WATCH**	
YEAR ONE	**$$**	**PANTS, SHOES, OUTERWEAR**
$$$	**SUITS, SPORT JACKETS, BRIEFCASE**	

In year one of building your work wardrobe, you have the biggest need and the least amount of capital. What's the solution? Plan carefully and be smart about your expenditures. To put it in architectural terms, build out from the foundation of the suit and sport jacket. This is where the key investment belongs because you want all the possible quality and versatility you can afford in these items. Smart choices here will pay off for several years.

Don't waste your limited resources on ties or fancy watches, etc. Ties and shirts at this stage should be simple, and relatively inexpensive—expecially considering the beating they will take between long hours at work and dry-cleaning wear and tear. An expensive watch will just look inappropraite—you want your management to believe you need a raise, not the opposite.

$$	**SHIRTS, TIES, PEN**	
YEAR FIVE	**$$$**	**PANTS, SHIRTS, TIES, SHOES**
$$$$	**SUITS, SPORT JACKETS, OUTERWEAR, WATCH**	

By the fifth year of your career, your wardrobe foundation should be solid and you will have started building up the essentials. Suits and jackets are still the priority here because they cost the most and have the greatest versatility. You may also want to invest in a nice overcoat at this point because, although pricey, it should last you for years.

Likewise, an expensive watch would be a good investment at this stage of your career assuming you purchase something that can last you until retirement. If you want to splurge on shirts or ties, make sure they are for special occasions—public speaking, important dinners—and that you treat them carefully. Good shoes will take a beating, of course, but by now you should have several pairs so you can rotate them. Now is the time to start investing in quality, rather than quantity.

The Ten...

It worked for Moses, it even works for David Letterman. There is something comforting about having some heads-up guidelines in lots of ten to help make sense of complicated subjects such as civilization or late-night TV. Obviously the bigger challenge is in figuring out what goes with what at 7 in the morning, avoiding costly mistakes by buying what either your significant other or saleperson gushes over, and, in general, just dressing yourself every day to avoid embarrassment. In light of the sheer magnitude of this we offer these thirty commandments...

LAWS OF DRESSING

1. You don't have to spend a lot on clothes to look like you've spent a lot.
2. Dark colors will always look more authoritative.
3. Classics are classics for a reason.
4. Dressing appropriately is like having good manners.
5. A tie should always be tied and in place, not worn half mast.
6. Nobody sees the label.
7. Quality is more important than quantity.
8. When in doubt, wear navy.
9. Or gray.
10. Clothes don't make the man. (Though they can fake the man.)

TIPS OF SMART SHOPPING

1. Dress appropriately for the stores you will be shopping in.
2. Wear a white dress shirt, dress socks, and the shoes you would wear for the outfit.
3. Always try things on.
4. Always look in the mirror (preferably a three-way mirror).
5. If it doesn't look good in the store, it won't look good at home.
6. There's nothing wrong with the lights in the store.
7. When something is on sale, don't buy it unless you would have bought it at full price (if you could have afforded it).
8. Something that's a little big can be tailored to fit. Something that's tight will only get tighter.
9. Shoes don't stretch.
10. The salesperson is supposed to tell you it looks great on you.

DEADLY SINS

1. Jackets that are too tight in the shoulders, snug in the waist, and won't button make you look like a trussed turkey.
2. Wear socks to the office, unless you work at the beach.
3. Just because it looked good on you ten years ago, doesn't mean it still does (refer back to deadly sin one).
4. Until you see the animals lining up in twos, don't have your pants tailored too short. They should have a break. Don't let your jacket be too short (your bottom line should never be visible).
5. Belts are to hold up your pants not some sort of technology tool holder. Pagers, phones and other digital elements belong in jacket pockets.
6. Pants that are too baggy look silly and pants that are too tight just look uncomfortable.
7. Wearing suspenders and a belt is redundant … and redundant.
8. You will look like a squeezed tube of toothpaste if your shirt is too tight in the collar.
9. Hoods on overcoats.
10. If you have to ask if it goes together, it probably doesn't.

Strategic Dressing
—Learning to Read the Landscape

"He was a self-made man who owed his lack of success to nobody."

JOSEPH HELLER
Catch-22

WHO LOOKS PROFESSIONAL AND WHAT ARE THEY WEARING?

One of the basic rules of office attire is: Dress for the job you want to have, not the job you have. So look around. Who has that job now? And how does he dress for that job? Now, who does he work for? And so on. Every office or corporation has a dress code. Learning to read yours properly is a major step toward getting ahead.

ALL DRESSED UP AND SOMEWHERE TO GO

Once you have cracked the office dress code, you have to consider what to wear for different professional occasions and situations. What may be appropriate for a morning meeting might not work for a business lunch or for a presentation. Begin by asking yourself what message you want to send and then find the appropriate clothes in your closet. Here are a few different scenarios:

Leading a meeting. Obviously what you're after here is authority, and nothing says authority like a suit. (After all, there's a reason why when people refer to management they call them "suits.") Since, in many offices, men remove their jackets while working, pay attention to the shirt you're wearing: Make sure it's crisp and clean.

Giving a presentation. When giving a presentation, you clearly want to have authority and draw attention to yourself. The key here is not to draw so much attention that you take away from the presentation. Once again, a suit is called for with a shirt and tie. And here is how

> "The first step toward getting somewhere is to decide that you are not going to stay where you are."
>
> **J. PIERPONT MORGAN**

you draw attention to yourself: With the tie. Without being too ostentatious or visually distracting, the shirt-and-tie combination should reflect power. Perhaps a shirt with French cuffs and a woven tie?

Client lunch. It is, of course, most important to come across as professional, but you must also be able to read the culture of the person (or people) you are meeting. Do they wear suits? Sport jackets? What about ties? The goal here is to be yourself but, at the same time, seem approachable. In other words, don't overpower the client by dressing more formally than they do; rather, show them the proper respect by dressing up more than you normally do if their corporate culture is more formal than yours.

Job review. This is just like a job interview so look your best. If you normally wear a suit to the office, do so now. If you don't usually wear one, doing so will only make you look stiff and feel uncomfortable. In that case, you should still dress up: Wear a sport jacket and tie. Show that you care, but don't look as though you're trying too hard.

Boss wants to have drinks. First of all, relax. It's only good. If you were in trouble, you would go to the boss, the boss wouldn't come to you. That said, look sharp. Yes, it's a social situation, but dress professionally and responsibly—and don't be afraid to show your personality. In other words, wear a tie that the boss might admire. Or a unique pair of cuff links that might spark a conversation. And don't drink too much.

shop smart

The suit you buy for your interview will not be the last one you ever buy, but since it may be the first one you own, it has to be versatile: Think of it as the Swiss Army knife in your closet.

How to Buy a Business Suit

WHAT DO I BUY FIRST?

Primary
- Suits
- Sport jackets
- Dress pants
- Dress shirts
- Ties

Secondary
- Chinos
- Sweaters
- Polo shirts
- Shoes
- Socks
- Belts
- Overcoats
- Accessories

SHOP SMART: PANTS

Color:
Dark gray = All business.
Black = Sophisticated, urban.
Tan = Earthy but sophisticated.
Fabric: For year-round, midweight wool and wool blends will get you through most seasons. In summertime, a tropical wool or linen is often more comfort-able, while in winter, a heavier wool or wool flannel will keep you better insu-lated.

Style: Again, the big decision here is whether to go with pleated or flat-front pants. Each is appropriate, but some larger men may find pleated trousers more roomy (although flat front is more slimming). Pleated pants should be cuffed ($1^1/2$") whereas flat-front trousers often look more streamlined when uncuffed. As for the width of the legs, styles vary slightly every season, but not enough so that it's noticeable. Basically, stay away from the extremes: Too narrow or too baggy. Most impor-tant, wear your trousers on your waist. You may think it's more comfortable to rest your pants below your gut, but it only highlights the fact that you have one. It just looks sloppy.

SHOP SMART: THE POLO SHIRT/SWEATER

What It Says: Although more casual than a shirt and tie, a nice polo sweater says you know how to work hard and still be comfortable.

How to Say It Best: A polo works best with a sport jacket, but it's refined enough to be paired with a suit. Navy and charcoal gray will mix best with your suits, while a maroon or dark green would likely go well with the sport jackets.

SHOP SMART: BRIEFCASES

Soft Briefcase: The soft briefcase (especially one with a convenient shoulder strap) has replaced the hard case in the last decade.

How to Say It Best: A soft leather briefcase should also be black, dark brown, or tan with either brass or silver fixtures.

The Attaché Case: This traditional hard case tells people you're all business—nothing is going to get in the way of your work, even if you have to lock it up.

How to Say It Best: Black, brown, or tan leather with brass or silver fixtures.

GOALS

Three or four suits, several sport jackets and pants, many shirts and ties, a few pairs of shoes, and a handful of power accessories.

Why It Matters: Building the proper business wardrobe is critical to success in the workplace as it prepares you for every occasion and signals to everyone that you belong.

Guidelines: What do I need? How much do I need?

Quality Control: At this point in your professional life, buy the best you can afford for your budget. It will certainly affect the quantity of what you purchase, but in the long run, the quality items will last longer and give you a greater return on the investment.

HALF WINDSOR

In this stage of your career, you have added some shirts and ties for special occasions.
With a spread collar and slightly richer and thicker tie, a half windsor makes a nice knot.
However, it should be an accent, not an everyday event—P.M. over A.M.

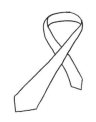 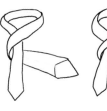 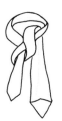 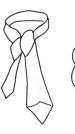 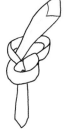 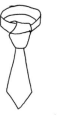 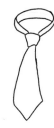

1. Begin with the tie's wide end approximately one foot below the narrow end, and cross it over the narrow end, bringing it back underneath.

2-3. Take the wide end up through the loop and pass it around the front from left to right.

4. Bring it through the loop again and pass it through the knot in front.

5. Tighten the knot slowly as you draw it up to the collar.

Work Wardrobe

As you begin to flourish in the workplace, your wardrobe must expand along with you. Always consider the atmosphere of your office, what your position is, and the long-term goals you have as you choose your business attire. And remember that what you see on the following pages needn't be accumulated immediately or even over one year. A wardrobe, like a career, takes time to build.

"The whole secret of a successful life is to find out what it is one's destiny to do, and then do it."

HENRY FORD

DO MY CLOTHES MEAN BUSINESS?

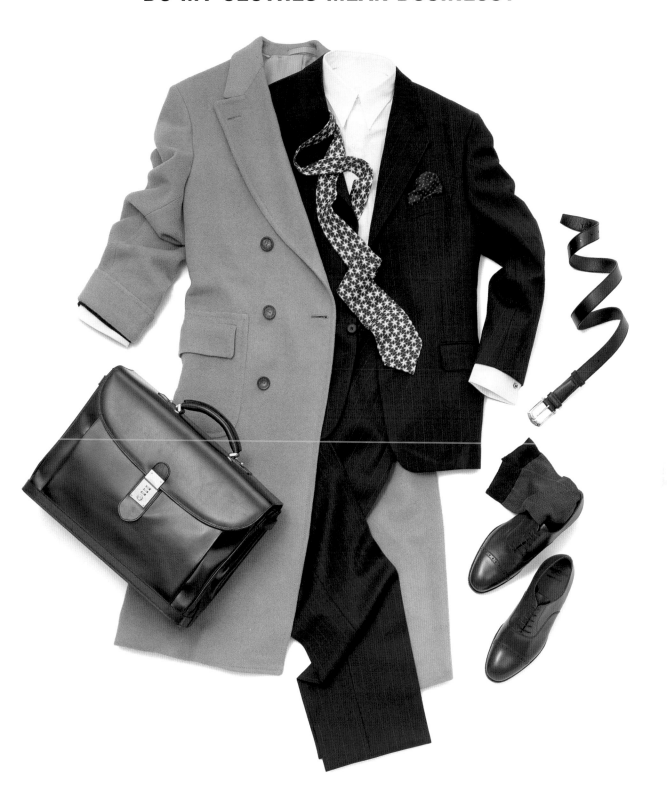

Navy Interview Suit + 3 Suits = Work Wardrobe

As with your interview suit, the suits you buy should be the best quality you can afford in classic styles. Following these guidelines will allow you versatility and will make your budget go further.

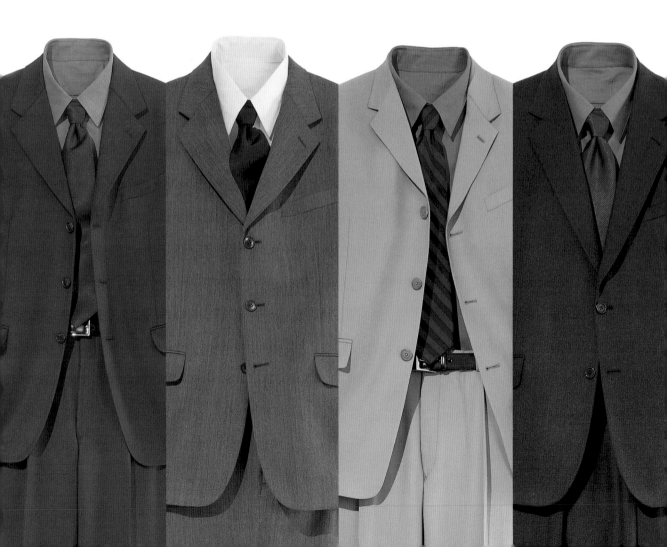

Dark Gray Suit

Just like a navy suit, gray is basic but vital. Everything looks good with gray and everything mixes with it. The fabric should be a worsted wool that can be worn nearly all year-round. A two- or three-button style is best (three-button is just as traditional and can often be more slimming), either with a single rear vent or without.

The world, of course, is not black and white, it's gray—and with good reason. It's elegant and formal. A man in gray is serious and unassailable. The tailoring on this suit should be the same as with the navy suit. Make sure the trousers are cuffed, and if they have little buttons on the inside of the waist, they're for suspenders.

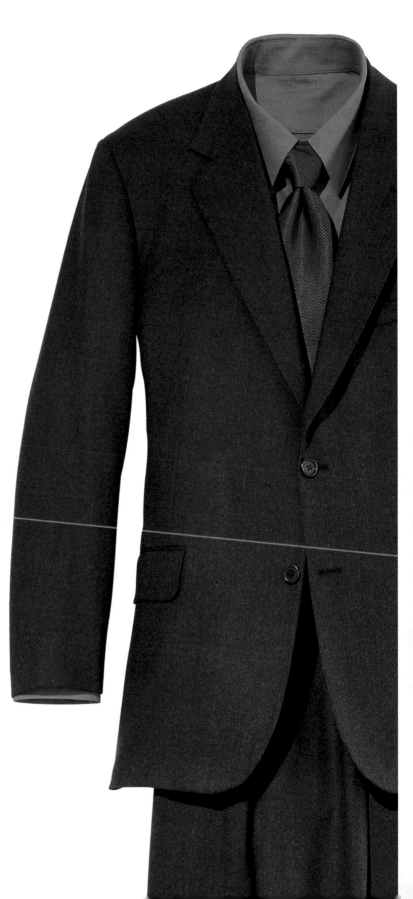

Light Gray Suit

For a third suit, light gray is a smart option. It is just as versatile as its darker cousin, and can be worn further into the summer months. A khaki suit is an alternative for this as well.

Opt for some variation between your gray suits. For instance, if the dark one is two-button, make this one three.

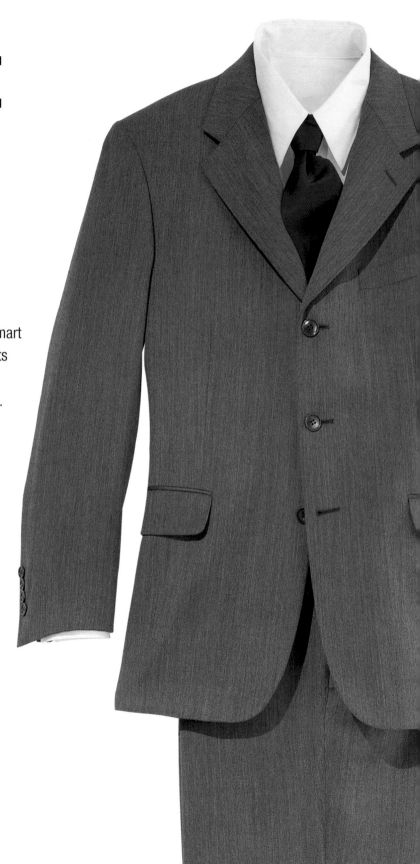

Khaki Poplin Suit

A warm weather essential for any man, the khaki suit is like navy for the summer. Split this suit in half when on the road and you have a pair of khaki pants or a khaki jacket.

The khaki suit is slightly more casual than darker suits, but it's still a suit. Dressy and polished, poplin is also lightweight, which makes it ideal for summer. Because the fabric is so lightweight, be sure the suit is pressed (or at least steamed) often. Otherwise, you can look like an unmade bed.

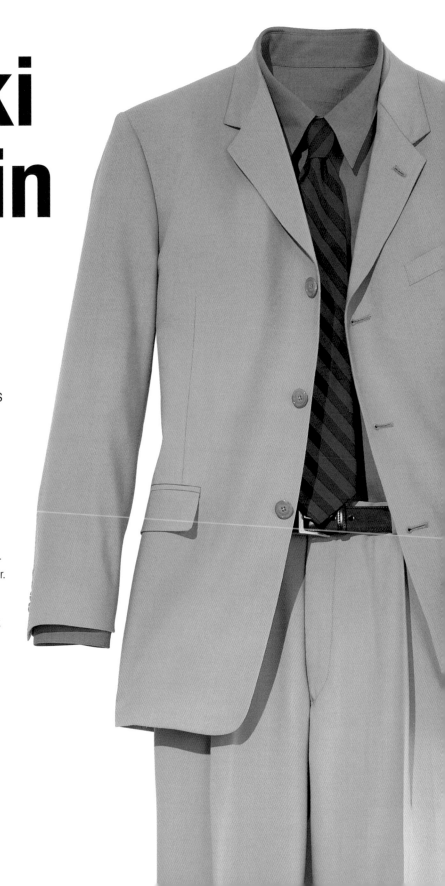

Bulletproof

The most formal sport jacket there is, a blazer is appropriate in any work environment and arguably the hardest-working item in your closet. A blazer with a little bit of structure in the shoulders and lining will fit more like a suit jacket than a more casual coat. Traditionally, the blazer has gold buttons (it began as a nautical uniform), but almost any store will offer dark navy buttons as well, or replace them free of charge. Go for this option: You're not Thurston Howell III.

The Blue Blazer

The blue blazer is like the remote control: Quite simply, no man can live without one. Perfect for the office, business lunches, travel, and weekends, a blazer can dress you up and take you anywhere. As with your suits, try to get a wool blazer that's light enough for summer and heavy enough for winter. Two-button single-breasted is best, but three-button is perfectly acceptable.

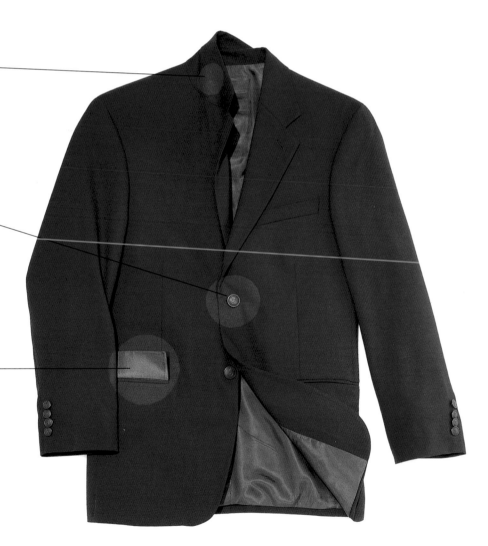

COLLAR
The collar of a jacket or suit should be lined with wool. This will help it lie flat against the neck and shoulders.

BUTTONS
Look for quality stitching around the buttons, meaning the thread is wrapped around itself many times to anchor them.

POCKETS
The pockets should be lined with rayon or cotton. This will help the jacket maintain its shape better. To ensure this even more, don't open your jacket pockets.

Sport Jackets

When a suit isn't called for, a sport jacket is. While not as dressy, it is certainly appropriate for the workplace. Indeed, as dress codes for the workplace have relaxed over the years, the sport jacket has become not only acceptable, but necessary; it provides flexibility and credibility. Paired with nice trousers and a shirt and tie (and sometimes without one), the sport jacket still looks extremely polished.

TESTING PATTERNS

Many patterned jackets trace their origin to the hunting and fishing pastimes of Scotland, which explains the names of those sporting-inspired designs: Houndstooth, herringbone, etc. Sport jackets provide an excellent opportunity to get some color, particularly earth tones, into your wardrobe. Since the patterns are often more casual looking, pay more attention to the tailoring to balance things out.

HERRINGBONE

An excellent way to begin with patterns because it's tweedy without being stuffy. The chevron design comes in large and small, but smaller is subtler, and therefore preferable.

HOUNDSTOOTH

Like herringbone, houndstooth comes in large and small variatons and, again, smaller is better. Black-and-white is classic, but shades of brown are no less traditional.

CHECK

Whereas houndstooth is more ragged (but not ragged-looking), the square check is neater and usually more bold.

PLAID

In a suit, plaid (sometimes known as a Prince of Wales plaid) can be formal, but in a sport jacket it's, well, sportier. Here, variations of brown are more versatile than black-and-white.

TWEED

Whether flecked or heathered, a simple tweed adds color and texture to your wardrobe. And unlike some of the other patterns, a tweed is more seasonal, ideal for cold weather.

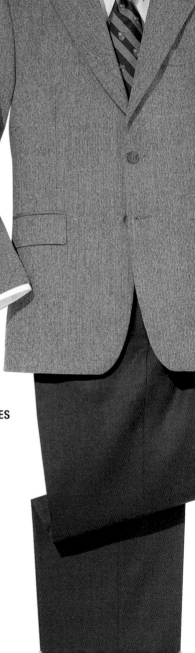

POWER OF SEPARATES
Herringbone Jacket
Button-Down Shirt
Striped Tie
Flannel Pants

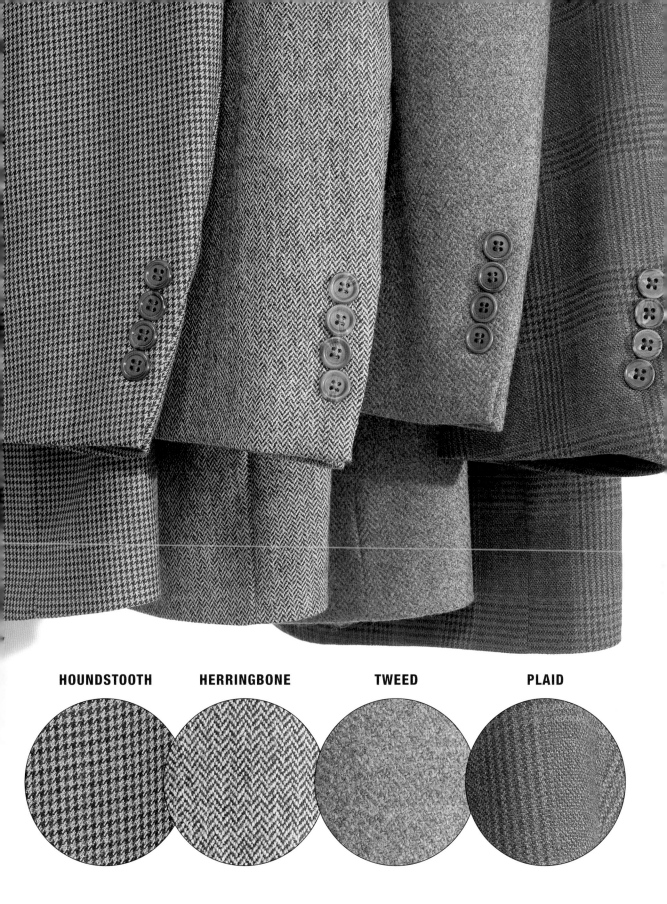

HOUNDSTOOTH

HERRINGBONE

TWEED

PLAID

Pants

PLEATED

FLAT-FRONT

Don't think trousers say much about a man? Then consider what the axiom "who wears the pants" is really asking: Who has the power? Unlike jeans or casual pants, dress slacks should be made of wool or wool blend, should never be wrinkled, and if treated properly will last for years. Since you will now be combining them with your sport jackets, think about what colors and materials will mix best and most often. As for the fit, if they're a bit tight in the waist now, they will only get tighter. And keep in mind that many trousers now have some stretch material in them. If you're wearing pants with stretch, less is more: Your colleagues should not be able to determine whether you're wearing boxers or briefs.

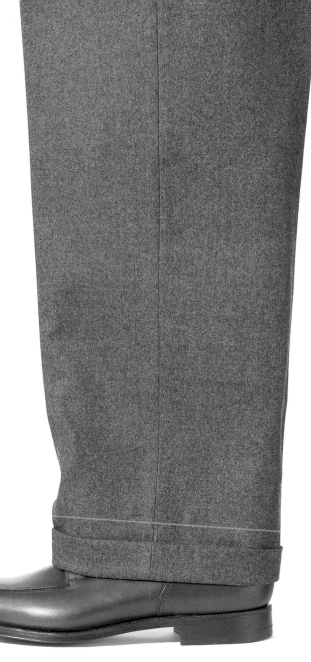

FLANNEL/WOOL/HEAVY FABRIC
DETAIL: Slightly more distinct, allows fabric to puddle slightly.
CUFFS: Flannel/wool/heavy fabrics/pleats.
BREAK: A subtle break just above the ankle helps the trousers drape better.

COTTON/WORSTED WOOL/LIGHTER FABRIC
DETAIL: Light break, cleaner line.
NO CUFFS: Flat-front/tuxedos/light fabrics.
BREAK: A very light break allows for a cleaner line and gives the appearance of more length.

POINT BREAK

Casual Pants

For days when you don't have to wear dress pants, nothing is more practical than chinos or khakis. (Despite the different names, these are actually the same thing.) Whether khaki or dark brown (yes, khakis can come in colors other than khaki), lightweight or heavy, chinos are all-purpose pants. But just because they're more casual doesn't mean they shouldn't look sharp. Don't wear anything with lots of visible external pockets or buttons (such as cargo pants), and always remember to have a crease in the legs. It will dress up even the most casual pants.

KHAKIS

Originally a work pant, they were a traditional "casual" choice for summer Fridays in the office. Dockers™ revolutionized the work dress culture by becoming the de facto choice of the new "gold rush" prospectors in Silicon Valley. Khakis are still a very valid choice but the key is well-pressed and sharp—let's not forget they come out of the spit-and-polish world of the military.

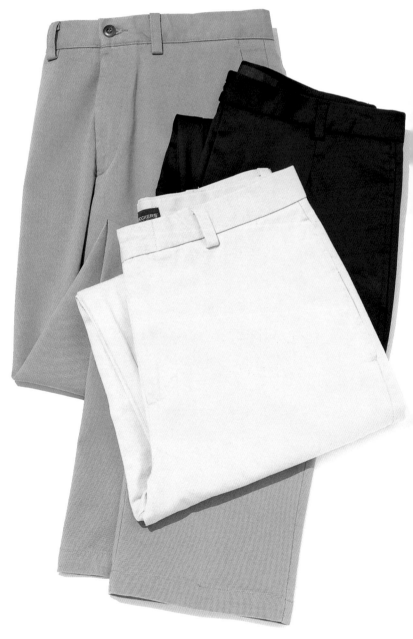

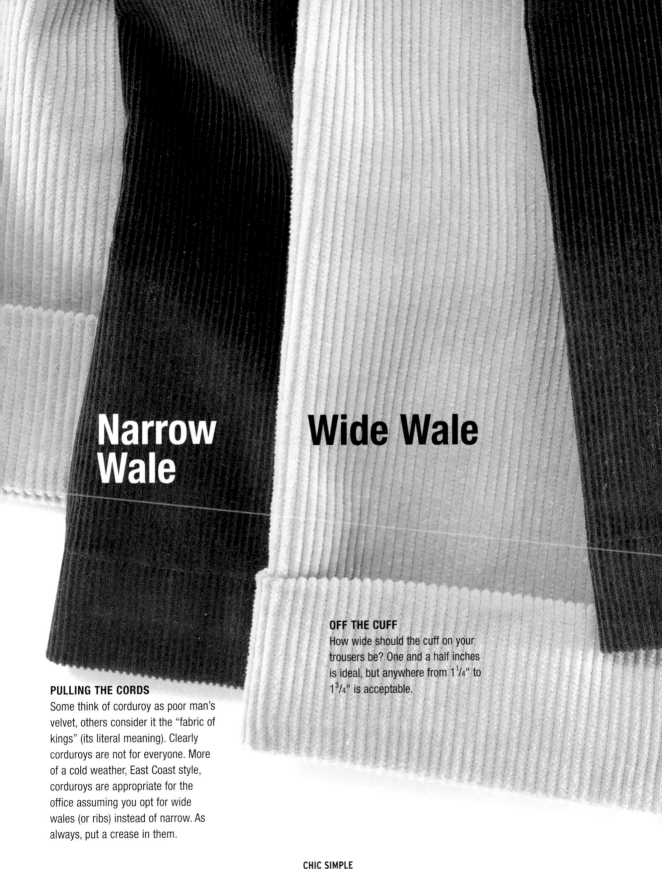

Narrow
Wale

Wide Wale

OFF THE CUFF
How wide should the cuff on your
trousers be? One and a half inches
is ideal, but anywhere from $1\frac{1}{4}$" to
$1\frac{3}{4}$" is acceptable.

PULLING THE CORDS
Some think of corduroy as poor man's
velvet, others consider it the "fabric of
kings" (its literal meaning). Clearly
corduroys are not for everyone. More
of a cold weather, East Coast style,
corduroys are appropriate for the
office assuming you opt for wide
wales (or ribs) instead of narrow. As
always, put a crease in them.

Shirt & Tie Wardrobe

As you start to build your shirt collection, variation is critical. Different fabrics, collars, and styles can make even the most basic shirts (white and blue) seem unique. Also, as you add patterns, be cognizant of what will mix well with your jackets and ties.

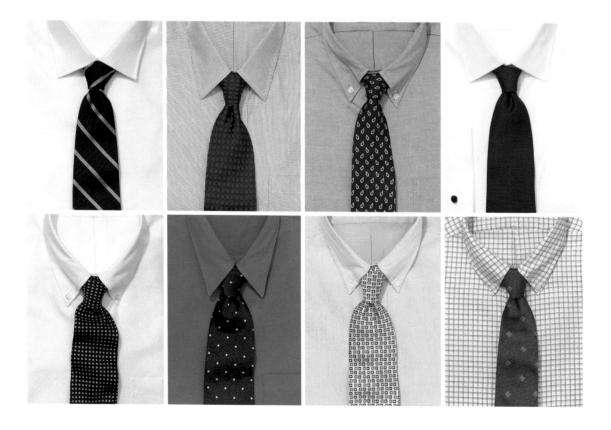

Button-Down

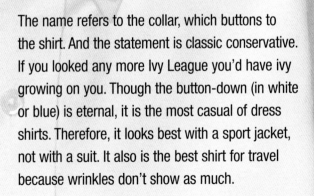

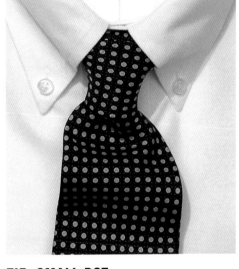

TIE: SMALL DOT

TIE: TONAL

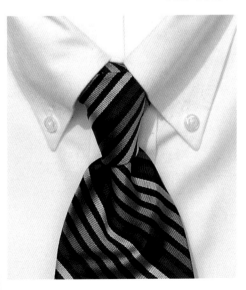

The name refers to the collar, which buttons to the shirt. And the statement is classic conservative. If you looked any more Ivy League you'd have ivy growing on you. Though the button-down (in white or blue) is eternal, it is the most casual of dress shirts. Therefore, it looks best with a sport jacket, not with a suit. It also is the best shirt for travel because wrinkles don't show as much.

Spread Collar

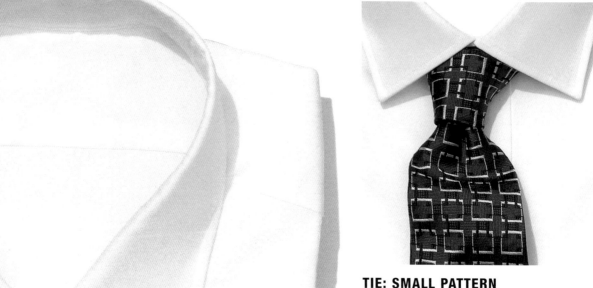

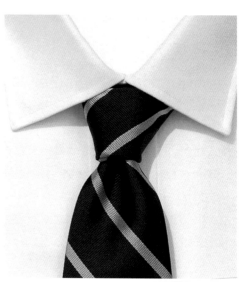

TIE: SMALL PATTERN

TIE: REP

Once thought of as a European-style shirt, the spread collar is now an American staple. Made of broadcloth, it gives a little more polish to a suit and tie. This shirt style looks best on men with thin faces as it will give the appearance of width.

Point Collar

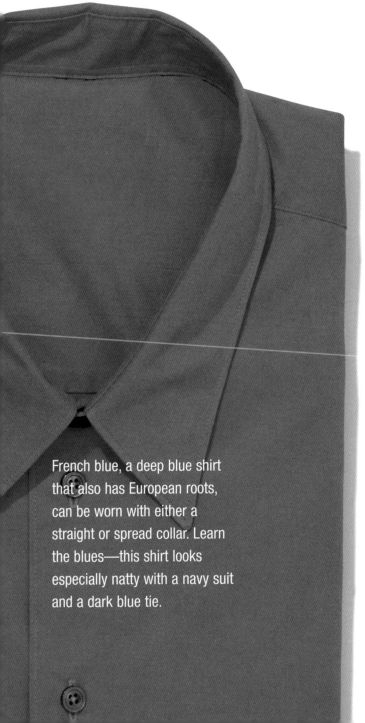

French blue, a deep blue shirt that also has European roots, can be worn with either a straight or spread collar. Learn the blues—this shirt looks especially natty with a navy suit and a dark blue tie.

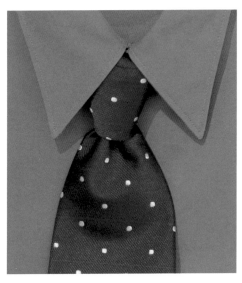

TIE: SMALL DOT

TIE: TEXTURED

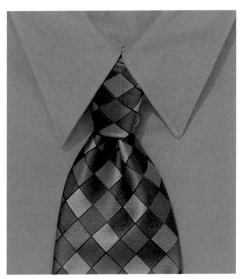

SHIRT & TIE
Oxford Cloth

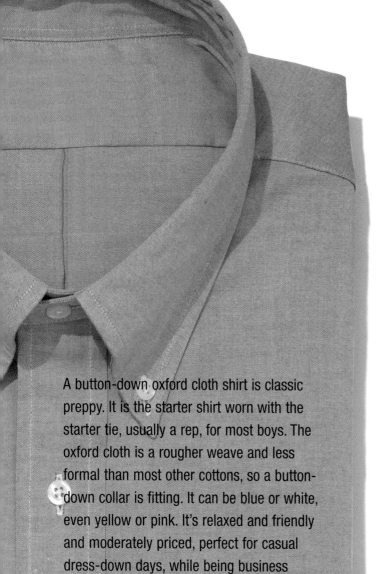

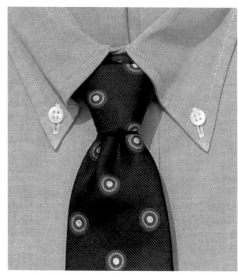

TIE: CLUB

TIE: PAISLEY

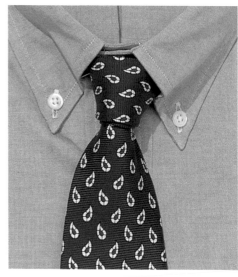

A button-down oxford cloth shirt is classic preppy. It is the starter shirt worn with the starter tie, usually a rep, for most boys. The oxford cloth is a rougher weave and less formal than most other cottons, so a button-down collar is fitting. It can be blue or white, even yellow or pink. It's relaxed and friendly and moderately priced, perfect for casual dress-down days, while being business appropriate. Dress up with a tie and blazer. Keep away from formal suits or occasions.

SHIRT & TIE
Stripes

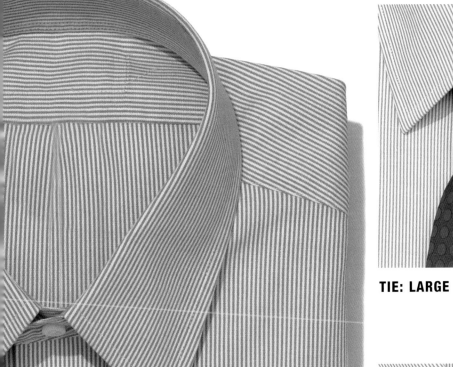

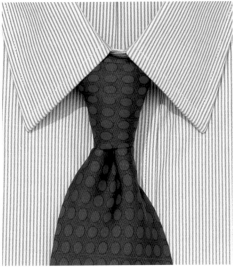

TIE: LARGE DOT

TIE: REP

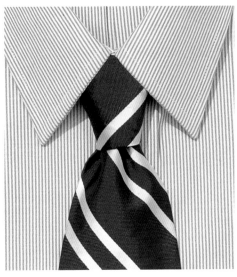

Shirts with thin, vertical stripes in one color are a business staple. The wider the stripe, however, the more eccentric the wearer. The same goes for multicolored striped shirts; anything more than two hues is a bit much. Pairing ties with striped shirts can be tricky at times. Solids are always safe. Striped ties work well as long as the stripes are bolder than those on the shirt. The same goes for patterns—they should be bolder than the stripe.

SHIRT & TIE
Color

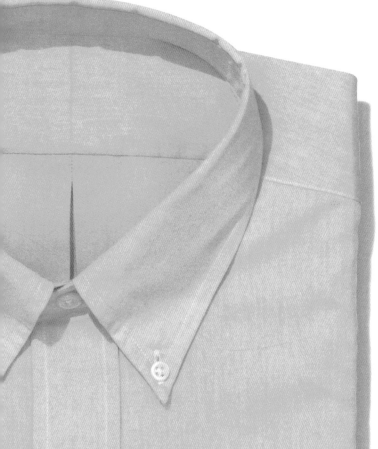

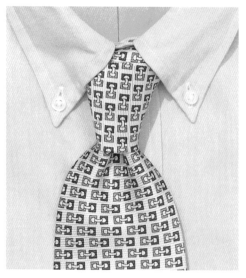

TIE: PATTERN

TIE: REP

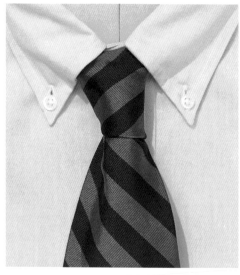

Color is an excellent way to break out of the monotony of white and blue. For now, light pastels—pink, yellow, purple, even green—are the safe way to go. They express individuality without being gaudy. Since the shirt is already adding a splash of color, try not to overpower it with an equally colorful tie. And be careful not to clash colors—say, a bright red with a pink.

SHIRT & TIE
Pattern

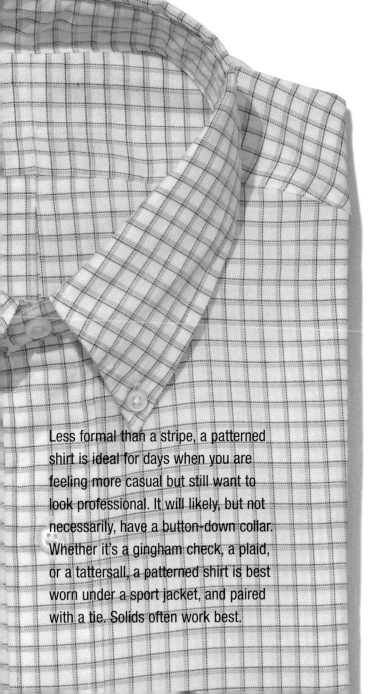

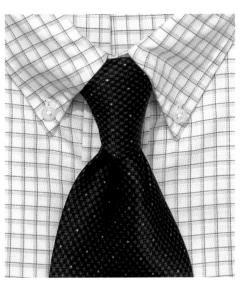

TIE: TEXTURED

TIE: SMALL PATTERN

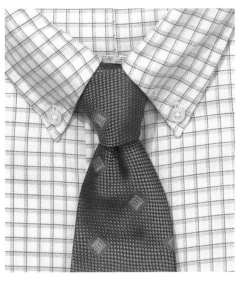

Less formal than a stripe, a patterned shirt is ideal for days when you are feeling more casual but still want to look professional. It will likely, but not necessarily, have a button-down collar. Whether it's a gingham check, a plaid, or a tattersall, a patterned shirt is best worn under a sport jacket, and paired with a tie. Solids often work best.

SHIRT & TIE
French Cuff

No dress shirt is as formal as white with French cuffs. Unlike those with barrel (or button) cuffs, shirts with French cuffs require cuff links. They come with straight or spread collars. This shirt looks best with a suit, though it can be worn with a sport jacket. Either way, save it for lunch with the boss.

KNOTTY BUT NICE
The best pair of first cuff links is a set of navy silk knots. Simple yet elegant (and very inexpensive), they come in almost every color and color combination.

HOW TO: CUFF LINKS
When putting on silk knots, start inside and work out. When putting on cuff links, align button holes, then start at the top and work down. Or call for help.

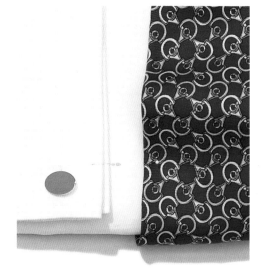

TIE: SMALL PATTERN
CUFF LINK: SILVER OVAL

TIE: SOLID
CUFF LINK: SILK KNOT

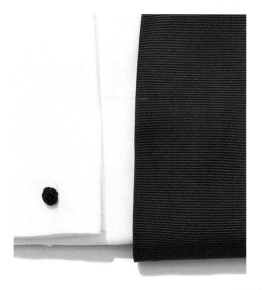

Polos

For those who can dress down (somewhat) at the office, a polo shirt or sweater is a smart option. With the advent of casual Fridays, it became a new classic. In cold weather, a long-sleeve merino polo is ideal (you can also put a white, navy, or black T-shirt underneath one), and in warmer climates, a smooth knit polo with a longer collar works best.

WORD TO THE WISE
Save those pique polos (those with nubby cotton fabric) for the weekends. They are too laid-back for the office.

Sweaters

A sweater at the office is really only needed in cold weather climates, but in some workplaces it may be acceptable office attire without a jacket. If you're wearing it with a jacket, merino wool is the most lightweight and shouldn't affect the fit of the coat. (Nor should a slightly heavier cashmere vest.) V-neck is better than crew neck, especially if you are wearing a tie. Charcoal and navy would be the colors to start with, and in general, sweaters go best with sport jackets not suits.

BLACK V-NECK MERINO SWEATER
WHITE SHIRT
PAISLEY TIE
Following the rule of two solids and one pattern, this combination works well with a pair of gray flannel or black trousers. The simple pairing of black and white is offset by the burst of color and pattern in the tie.

NAVY V-NECK LAMB'S WOOL VEST
GINGHAM SHIRT
SOLID BLUE TIE
A dressed-up alternative for a casual Friday, this combination adds a bit of polish (with the tie) to an otherwise relaxed shirt and sweater pairing. Note how the solid blue tie doesn't compete with the shirt. This could work well with a pair of gray or tan trousers and a blue blazer.

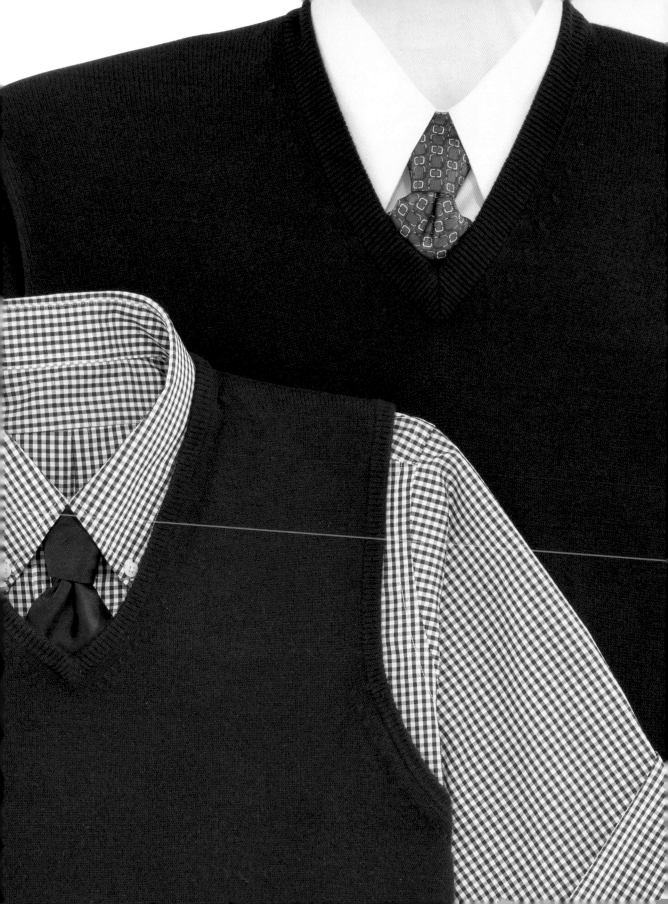

Shoes &

Nothing takes a greater beating than your shoes. Having more shoes, while expensive, means you will be wearing them out more slowly. Rotating your shoes will help them last longer.

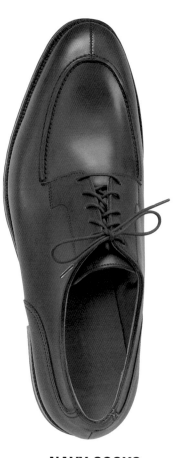

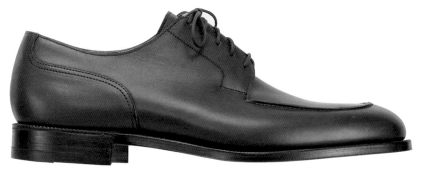

BROWN SPLIT-TOE LACE-UP
A proper dress shoe with style but not so much that you're seen as a dandy. These shoes will look best with your brown and gray pants. If you're feeling confident, try them with the blue suit. But no matter what, never match them with black socks. (Note: These shoes can also be worn in black.)

NAVY SUIT

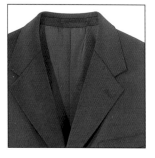

+

BROWN SHOES

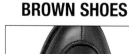
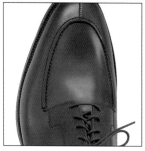

=

NAVY SOCKS

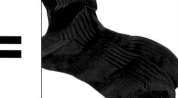

BROWN PANTS

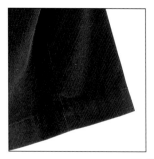

+

BROWN SHOES

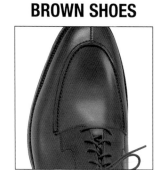

=

NAVY/BROWN SOCKS

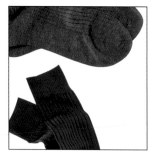

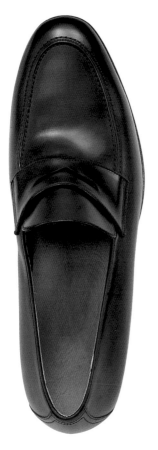

Socks

Dress socks should be made of wool or cotton. Be careful when matching them—black and blue look a lot alike, especially in the A.M., and you may go to work wearing one of each. At least you'll have a matching pair at home.

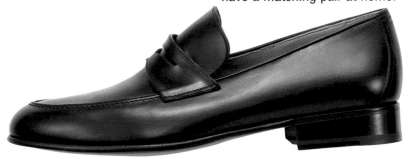

BLACK LOAFERS

Like the oxford shirt, penny loafers are a classic, but a casual classic. Because the loafer is more casual than a lace-up shoe, it looks better with a sport jacket than with a suit. Oh, and people stopped putting pennies in them in second grade.

GRAY PANTS

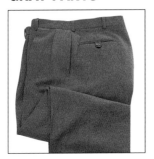

+

BLACK LOAFERS

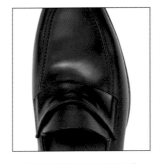

=

BLACK/GRAY SOCKS

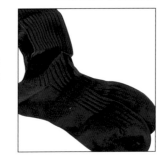

KHAKI PANTS

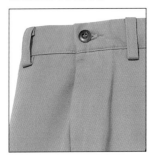

+

BLACK LOAFERS

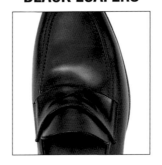

=

BLACK SOCKS

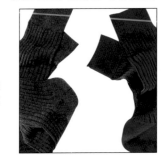

Coats

Just because you're not in the office doesn't mean you shouldn't look professional. (What, you never run into a colleague on the street?) There are two items you need to start building your outerwear wardrobe, and each will get the right message across through rain or sleet or…

TRENCH COAT

MACKINTOSH

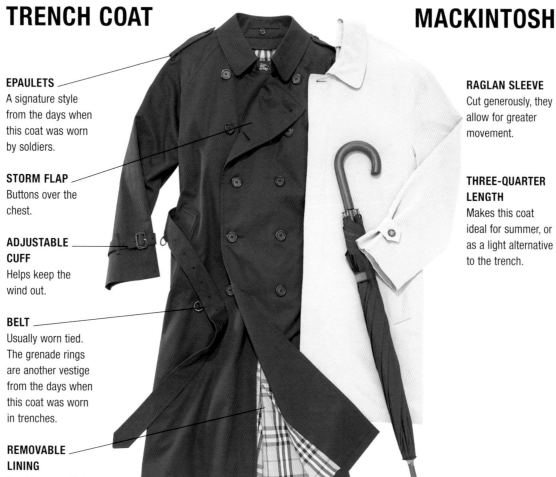

EPAULETS
A signature style from the days when this coat was worn by soldiers.

STORM FLAP
Buttons over the chest.

ADJUSTABLE CUFF
Helps keep the wind out.

BELT
Usually worn tied. The grenade rings are another vestige from the days when this coat was worn in trenches.

REMOVABLE LINING
Provides warmth in winter and keeps the coat light enough for summer.

RAGLAN SLEEVE
Cut generously, they allow for greater movement.

THREE-QUARTER LENGTH
Makes this coat ideal for summer, or as a light alternative to the trench.

UMBRELLA

Keep that small, collapsible umbrella in your desk or briefcase for emergencies, but for every day get a classic, full-sized black umbrella with a wooden handle. Not only will it keep you drier, but it will also fit more people underneath—like, say, your boss.

TRENCH COAT

This foul-weather staple is eminently businesslike. A removable lining will make it a year-round article. With a classic khaki trenchcoat, single-breasted is ideal for younger guys; double-breasted works best on older men. If you like the double-breasted trench, black is tough-looking without seeming like you're Sam Spade.

MACKINTOSH

Named for the Scottish chemist, Charles Macintosh, who invented the process of rubberizing fabric to make it waterproof, the Mackintosh raincoat is a lighter alternative to the traditional trench coat. In a three-quarter length, the Mac is ideal for summer.

OVERCOAT

The style of the coat should relate to the style of the jacket. In other words: A single-breasted navy or gray wool coat with notch lapels. Accessories are just as important outside of the office. To complement the overcoat, consider a lamb's wool scarf (in navy, charcoal, or red) and a pair of black leather gloves.

OVERCOAT

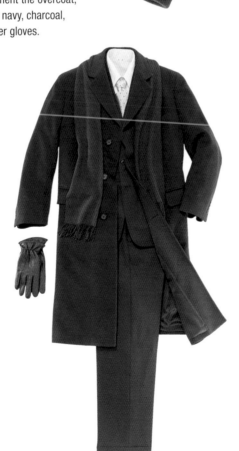

LINING

The rayon or silk lining helps ease movement.

WOOL SCARF

A gray, blue, or reddish lamb's wool scarf will keep your neck and chest warm.

LEATHER GLOVES

A stylish way to finish off the look. Lined with lamb's wool.

Tools of the

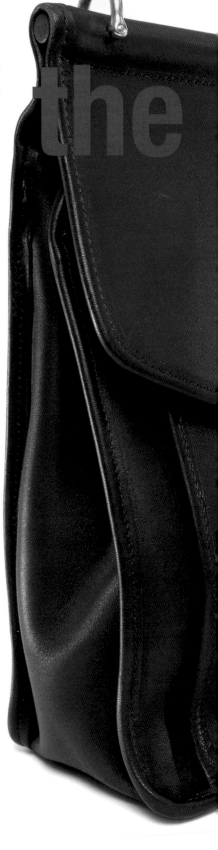

BRIEFCASE VS. KNAPSACK

Alas, you stopped carrying a Scooby-Doo lunch box at one point in your life (you have stopped, haven't you?), and now it's time to abandon the knapsack in favor of a briefcase. Infinitely more stylish and far more grown-up, a briefcase is a sign that you are ready to be serious about your career. Choose one in black or brown leather and make sure there's enough room to grow but not bulge. Be sure there is reinforced stitching on stress points, not too many pockets (shrinks the available space), and a light interior color (easier to spot lost objects).

THE WRITE STUFF

Seeing as how mighty the pen is, it makes sense to carry one with some impact. You never know when you'll be called on to hand it over to someone more senior or sign something important in public. Get yourself a nice metal pen (with a hard point as opposed to a felt tip) and be quick on the draw when someone in authority asks for one.

MONEY CLIP

Want something lighter than a wallet? Consider a money clip (made of brass or silver). Assuming you don't cram every receipt, photo, and credit card you own in there—and now is the time to DeJunk—it's a streamlined way to go.

WHAT'S ON YOUR AGENDA

A smart businessman keeps his appointments and is always on time. The first step to doing that is maintaining an agenda. Whether it's a small leather note-book with dates and addresses or a high-tech PDA, a well-maintained agenda will bail you out time and time again.

MONEY MATTERS

Anything that someone in the workplace might see affects your appearance—and that includes your wallet. After all, you might have to pay for a business lunch some day and you can't be pulling out that old Velcro number from seventh grade. So, as with belts and briefcases, stay with black or brown leather. Also, try keeping your wallet in your jacket's breast pocket so it doesn't get bent out of shape.

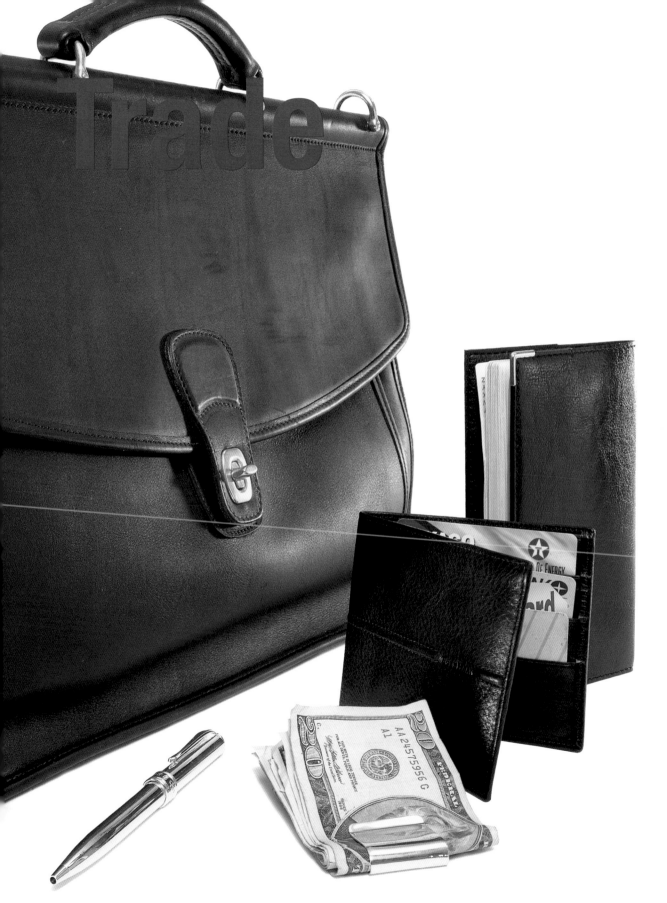

CLOSET work wardrobe

Your refrigerator is probably stocked, but is your closet? Take a moment to consider what you need, and whether what you have is meeting your career goals. Below is a checklist for the first year on the job and the fifth. It's just a guideline, but if you follow it, you should be set for years to come. Your goals: To create a flexible work wardrobe so that: 1. You never have to wear the same outfit twice in one week, and 2. You will look appropriate in any work environment.

FIRST-YEAR CHECKLIST

2 or 3 suits
1 or 2 sport jackets
7–10 dress shirts
3 or 4 pairs of pants
2 pairs of shoes
5–7 ties
1 briefcase

FIVE YEARS AND COUNTING

5–8 suits
4 or 5 sport jackets
6–8 pairs of pants
5 pairs of shoes
15–20 ties
3 sweaters

Your closet should now be filled with all of the clothes you need to get ahead in the workplace: Enough suits, shirts, ties, pants, shoes, and a few power accessories to get you through each season, all types of weather, and every occasion. And, because you purchased wisely, many of these clothes will last you for years to come.

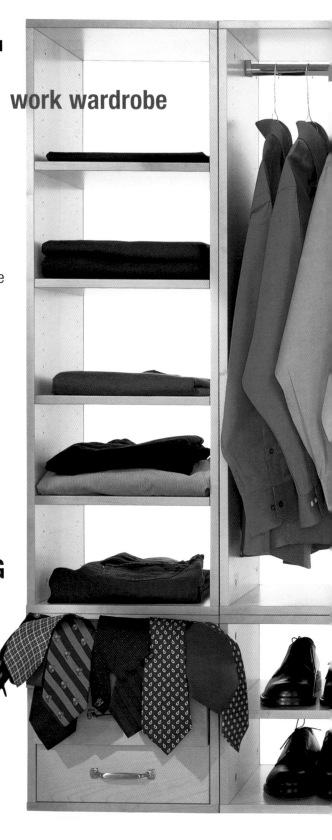

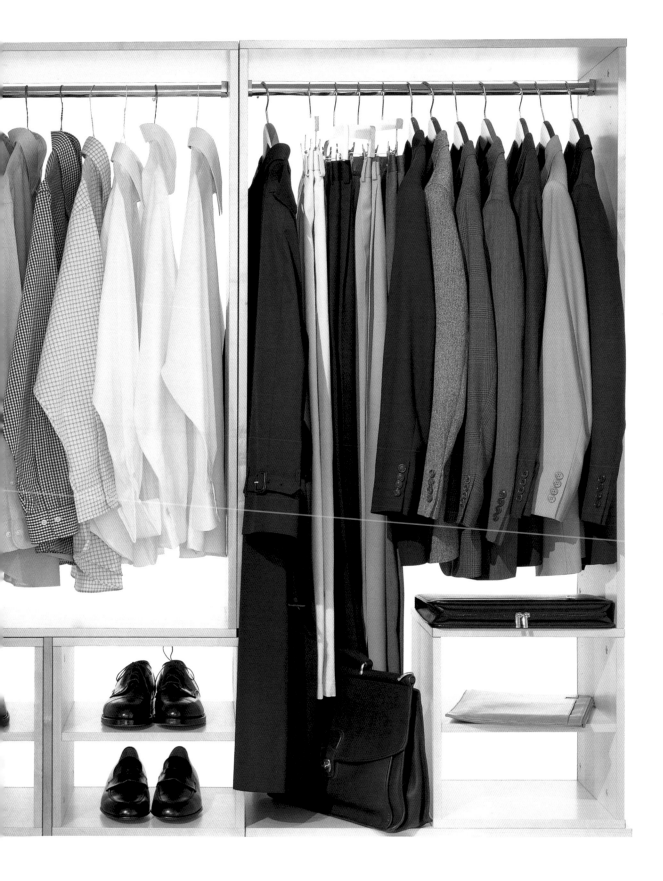

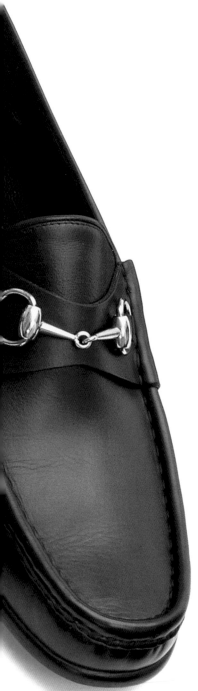

WHAT SUITS YOU?

Dear jeff and Kim,
I was just promoted to VP of my division, and travel a lot between Seattle and LA. I bought a black suit, but I'm not sure what to wear with it. I have a gray shirt and dark tie but I feel my lace-up oxfords aren't right. I sometimes think I look like I'm going to a funeral.
—Paint It Black

Dear Paint It Black,
Once fashion-forward, the black suit has become mainstream—a new classic. If you don't feel right in your lace-ups (which are fine by the way) then get a good pair of loafers. A black suit looks great with a French blue shirt and a dark tie, pattern or solid. A good suit is also great for after-work events with an open dress shirt, as well as occasions that are black tie optional. Translation: Don't wear a tux unless you are the waiter. A black suit, white shirt, and a silver or dark tie (if not black) create an evening outfit without the hoopla of a tuxedo.

—jeff and Kim

Get Better Job

3

Power Wardrobe

It was in *Wall Street* that Michael Douglas, as Gordon Gekko, got to rave "Greed works! Greed will save the USA!" It is safe to say that the character had a firm grasp on power as many know it. And he had the clothes to prove it. What is it that gives clothes an aura of power? Part of it is the cultural association to things such as movies—some of it is the ability to afford luxurious things. In the end, though, a sense of elegance comes from the taste and ability to dress in a timeless style that speaks of the individual. You may wear what you see in the movies, or a shirt a boss wears, or a suit of a business leader, but if it isn't you, then you're only wearing a costume—doing business in drag. The key is to slowly learn what makes you feel good and confident. With that you begin to create a wardrobe of personal style. Your uniform of self.

Dressing to Get Ahead

> "Power can corrupt, but absolute power is absolutely delightful."
>
> **ANONYMOUS**

WHO'S IN CHARGE HERE?

After several years on the job, you have likely been moving up—or else you're ready to move out. If you've been racking up promotions, your wardrobe of the last few years needs to be improved on. It's not that it's no longer appropriate for work—look at all the successful junior people in the office, they're dressing like you now, aren't they?—it's just that you now need to dress with authority. You need to have a wardrobe with some power.

To get where you want to go takes a lot of hard work, and your wardrobe has been a part of your climb up the ladder. Now, more than ever, as you seek a better position (whether inside your company or out), this aphorism is essential: Dress for the job you want to have, not for the one you already have. In other words, if you're still dressing like a bit player, no one will ever see you as the leading man.

Of course, the mailroom clerk who dresses like a managing director will never get the job he seeks simply because he wears the right jacket and tie, but it might cause someone to think he's capable of that job some day. By the same token, if you're the managing director who dresses like a mailroom clerk, you are, perhaps, building a glass ceiling over your head.

Keep in mind, however, that you should dress one level above— don't try skipping three or four. Dressing for the next job only works if you don't upstage your superiors. They don't want you dressing better than they do.

CONSISTENCY—AVOIDING MIXED SIGNALS

Your employees look to you for guidance. If you dress commandingly every day, you will appear confident and secure, like the kind of man who has everything under control. Then, if you dress down on Fridays, you may be sending the message that everyone can relax a bit on that day.

Similarly, if you aspire to rising in the ranks, be aware that your big break could come at any moment, so dress accordingly.

LOOKING LIKE A MILLION—WITHOUT MAKING A MILLION

One of the many perks of climbing the ladder is greater financial security. And as you earn more money, you will find that you will likely spend more. Improving certain aspects of life—a better car, a new house, nicer vacations—is one of the many rewards of success. So, too, must you make a new investment in your wardrobe.

Becoming more successful, however, doesn't require that you wear $2,000 suits (unless of course if you can afford them and appreciate them) but it doesn't really allow for $200 suits anymore, either. What you need to learn now is how to invest in quality.

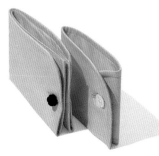

WRIST SHOTS
A double cuff that turns back and is usually fastened with a cuff link, the French cuff makes an elegant statement at the wrist. If you purchase a shirt with a contrasting collar and cuffs, the cuffs should always be French cuffs.

POCKET SQUARES VS. HANDKERCHIEFS

The pocket square—a piece of colored silk kept in your jacket breast pocket—comes in and out of style and is, at best, tricky. Never match your tie color, but keep it the same hue. A fine linen handkerchief folded or stuffed in your pocket is much safer. Below are two simple methods of handkerchief control.

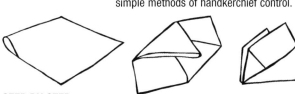

STEP BY STEP
The Triangle Fold

1. Fold the linen in quarters.

2. Fold the sides into the center.

3. Bend the bottom half backward and fold in half.

4. Place in pocket.

The Puffed Fold. Grab the center of the handkerchief and let it fall upside down, smooth with the other hand, gathering most of the material like a flower. Fold the center end under, and stuff neatly into pocket.

quality & quantity

There are clearly two ways to spend your money: Quantity and quality. As you seek a better position in your career, both are important. Quantity will give you more choices. If, for instance, you now have seven suits instead of four, you have more options, which will only make life easier when getting dressed or packing for travel. Quantity allows you to be more versatile in different situations: Whereas you once had only a blue blazer that was too heavy to wear in, say, summer, you will now have two blazers, one for warm weather and one for cold.

Quality, on the other hand, has more subtle value. Quality clothing may cost more, but it is also a kind of shorthand for status. Better clothes often send a faster signal to people that you know how to invest in yourself. The right watch, for instance, is a status symbol to many people, and wearing one that looks expensive tells people that you know more than what time it is. And keep in mind, it only needs to look expensive. A Timex, in other words, may go just as far as a Rolex.

How to Identify Quality

Another advantage of clothing that is well made is that it tends to last longer. The fabrics are more durable, the workmanship is finer, and so repairs are often easier. Think of it this way: Would you rather own an expensive car that was relatively easy to service or one that was medium-priced but a headache to fix?

THE SIGNS OF QUALITY

If the price tag is not a sign of quality—and let's be clear, it isn't—then what is? Quality comes in many forms, and understanding what to look for will help you become a smarter shopper and dresser.

QUALITY CUT

There is no single perfect cut of a suit. Single-breasted is not better than double. Having two buttons on your jacket is not any less valuable than three. Rather, the beauty of clothes lies in the eyes of the ultimate beholder: You. Understanding the most flattering cut of clothing for your body type is critical to seeking out quality.

Clothing can often make up for what nature has not given us. If you don't have broad shoulders, some padding in your suit jacket may give you a little more heft. If you are shorter than you would like, a lean-cut, vertically striped suit with three buttons will give you the appearance of length. A little heavy in the middle? Try darker suits without a vent in the rear. The point is, what you are looking for is relative to who you are and what you look like.

The next step is understanding what designers and labels are most ideal for you. Some jackets are boxier than others—heavier men would want to avoid these. Some are cut narrow in the shoulders, and men with broad chests would be wise to steer clear. Even if you have always coveted owning a certain name-brand designer's clothes, they may not be well suited for your shape and size, and it would be wiser to spend your money on something that fits better. After all, you don't wear the label on the outside.

Once you have identified brands that are tailored for your body, that is your quality cut. Again, it may not be right for your best friend, your father, or your younger brother, but a quality cut only has to suit you.

QUALITY FABRIC

All fabrics are not created equal. If they were, you could wear a pair of silk pants to play touch football in—and good luck with your friends on that one—and a denim tie to the office. But how a fabric looks is often not as important as how it feels. A fabric's feel or finish will affect not only how good you look in an article of clothing, but also how it feels to have it on. As a rule,

heavier fabrics are usually more durable while the quality fabrics feel better and are more fragile.

Suits and Jackets. That first suit you wore on an interview was a worsted wool. Nothing wrong with it, of course (in fact it holds a crease quite well), but it's just not as luxurious feeling—or looking—as a Super 100 wool (which refers to the fineness of the fibers themselves). Nor does it drape as well or stay unwrinkled quite like a wool crepe (which refers to how it is woven together). Cashmere, while incredibly soft to the touch and very warm, is a bit too heavy for suits. It is, however, ideal for, say, a blue blazer or, better yet, an overcoat.

Shirts. The first shirts you owned were broadcloth or oxford cloth, two cottons that feel very nice, but they aren't nearly as soft as Egyptian cotton or Sea Island cotton, which have a higher thread count per square inch. In general, if you want to spend money on better fabrics, you should think about which fabrics will be close to the body: Shirts, pants, etc. After all, certain silk ties may feel better, but they're only going to feel good against your shirt.

Ties. As with wools and cottons, some silks are smoother than others. Such softer silks are said to have a finer "hand," a fact you can test with either your left or right. A necktie made of a finer silk will often look better tied (meaning the knot looks more defined or it holds a center dimple better), but it may also wrinkle faster and be ruined more quickly by, oops, that soup you just spilled.

Sweaters. As far as sweaters are concerned, Shetland is a basic, durable wool, as is lamb's wool. But neither feels as fine to the hand as merino, cashmere, or silk (all of which are often

combined in sweaters). But again, quality does matter even in these categories (all fabrics are not created equal, remember?). It would be wiser to buy an expensive merino V-neck than a more expensive cashmere sweater that was thin and cheap looking. After all, why buy a cashmere sweater that pills and looks ragged when you can have a smart-looking merino version for less money that will last longer?

Shoes. Nothing takes a beating like your shoes, so investing in quality materials is a risky concept. A supple leather, such as cordovan, will scratch more easily than one that is more rugged. A good suede can be ruined by the rain. And snow. And dirt. Still, because you are investing in quantity and quality, you have more shoes in your closet, so you can be judicious about when you wear the nicer ones.

QUALITY WORKMANSHIP

A man who kicks the tires of a car he's thinking of buying clearly knows nothing about quality—it's just not where you look. The same is true for clothing. It is only when you know where to look for quality that you can know if you're truly getting your money's worth. Quality workmanship often does not show. It is often hidden in subtle details such as stitching, lining, and construction. Handcrafted items are usually (but not always) better made than those processed on a machine. The stitching and construction are simply more reliable than on something that is mass-produced.

Suits and Jackets. There are many distinguishing signs of quality workmanship to look for in a suit or sport jacket. Here are a few that should make a difference: A jacket with internal construction will drape better across the body and will retain its shape longer. You can usually feel the support inside the shoulders and across the back of the jacket, and it might also feel slightly heavier than an unconstructed jacket, but not enough to weight you down. A lining in the pockets will protect them better, but the truth is, it's best never to open your jacket pockets; stuffing them with keys, change, and other effluvia will only cause the jacket to bulge and will distort its shape.

Buttons are another sign of quality. Good jacket buttons are made out of very hard plastic and sometimes even horn. On truly superior jackets, the buttons on a sleeve will actually work, and the buttonhole on a lapel will actually be a hole. With trousers, well-made pants will have several buttons in the inside of the waistband for suspenders.

Shirts. Stitching is what you're looking for here. A well-made shirt will have fine stitching down the placket (the material down the front where you button it), and across the yoke and shoulders. Look for about 14 stitches per inch on the placket. There will also be attention paid to the collar, perhaps the most critical part of a shirt. A well-constructed collar will retain its shape longer. And once again, buttons are the sign of workmanship. Mother-of-pearl buttons are among the best you can get, but a good, hard plastic that won't crack or chip is the least you should expect.

Ties. A well-made tie will have a lining (usually linen or wool) that extends to the tip of both ends. This will help it retain its shape after many wearings. A good tie should also have hand stitching along the back. Finally, look for a loop of fabric on the wide end to tuck the narrow end into when it's tied. This will preserve the tie better and keep you from tucking it into the label.

Shoes. Since shoes take the most punishment, great care must be paid to purchasing pairs that won't fall down on the job. Look for leather with a smooth finish; it will better resist cracking. The soles should be leather and be lightly tanned and flexible. A well-made shoe should not have upper parts that are glued; look for stitching or, if you don't have an eye for this, ask the salesman.

FULL WINDSOR

The full Windsor is a dinosaur of a knot that is mistakenly credited to the Duke of Windsor. Not only did the duke not invent this knot but he also didn't wear it, preferring instead the four-in-hand with very thick ties. It is just too big and no one wears it (including its namesake, not a good sign). However, you now have the secret knowledge to tie this classic knot. If you do want to try this out, wear it only with a wide spread English collar and when asked to attend royal weddings.

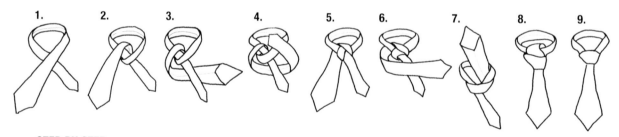

STEP BY STEP

1. Take the broad end of the tie in your right hand and pass it over the narrower end.
2. The broader end goes from under and around the narrow end.
3. Pull it over the knot and down toward your body through the loop that has been formed.
4. The broader end is now hanging down on the right, wrong side facing up.
5. Take the broader end and pass it around the half knot.
6. Take the thick end of the necktie and pass it up from below and behind the knot and through the loop around your neck.
7. Carefully pull the broader end over the half-completed knot.
8. Next, put the tip of the broad end underneath the outer layer of the knot.
9. Pull the broad end right through and carefully adjust the knot, holding it gently and pulling the narrower end.

HAND-STITCHING
At stress points strategic to fit (collar, sleeve), stitches will be visible beneath the collar at the back of the neck and around the inside armhole. The more stitches per inch, the better quality the tailoring.

LAPELS
Should lie perfectly flat without buckling.

POCKETS
Lined in cotton.

LINING
Silky Bemberg rayon, preferably full length.

FABRIC
Soft and pliant to the touch.

PATTERN
Should always line up without interruption across pockets and seams.

A CLOTHING CANVAS

Lesser-quality suits, and most that are ready-made, achieve contouring through fusing, or heat-welding the fabric at the risk of puckering. If the lapel feels like a single piece when you rub it between thumb and forefinger, a "fusible" has probably been used.

BUTTONHOLES

Irregular stitches around the buttonhole indicate, ironically, quality. They're evidence of hand-sewing.

SEAMS

In unconstructed jackets without a lining look for seams that are taped, without ragged edges. Double-faced fabrics obviate the need for a lining in this type of tailoring.

EXTERIOR POCKETS

On soft suits these pockets are often of the patch variety—a sportier pocket once found only on sport coats.

SHOULDER

A soft suit has only the lightest of padding in the shoulder to create an easy sloping line—a characteristic that allows it to be worn without its matching trousers (as long as you wear it with some sort of trousers).

INTERIOR POCKETS

Some suits do not have complete linings, therefore there are fewer interior pockets; but expect at least one for pen and wallet.

SLEEVE

Set without puckering to hang slightly forward, tapering gently from the shoulder to the hem; neither too tight nor too full. Even when the jacket is without lining, sleeves still need to be lined with a quality silk or rayon for ease of movement.

SINGLE-NEEDLE STITCHING

A more costly and time-consuming method of machine sewing that uses one needle to sew one side of a garment at a time, providing a consistent, careful stitch. The faster, less expensive method is to sew with double-needle stitching, working both sides of the garment at once, with a greater likelihood of puckering.

HAND-STITCHING

At stress points strategic to fit (collar, sleeve), stitches will be visible beneath the collar at the back of the neck and around the inside armhole. The more stitches per inch, the better quality the tailoring.

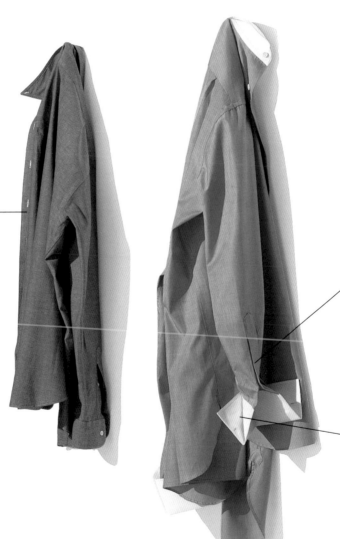

FIT

Sufficient blousiness in the sleeve. Where it joins the cuff, fabric should be gathered into pleats, not tapered.

PLACKET

A count of 14 stitches per inch on a shirt's placket—the strip of fabric on which the buttons are sewn—indicates quality. Fewer than 11 per inch signals lesser quality.

BUTTONS

Cross-stitched and made of mother-of-pearl.

LONG TAILS

Long enough to come together between the legs.

SPLIT-SHOULDER YOKE

A vertical seam down the yoke on the back of the shirt.

COLLAR

Evenly stitched around the edges.

GAUNTLET BUTTON

An anachronistic button on the sleeve opening, above the cuff.

FRENCH CUFFS

To be worn with cuff links.

1. POCKET DETAIL

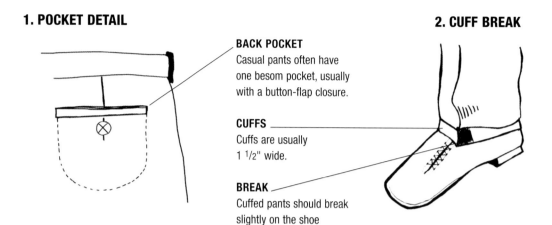

BACK POCKET
Casual pants often have one besom pocket, usually with a button-flap closure.

CUFFS
Cuffs are usually 1 1/2" wide.

BREAK
Cuffed pants should break slightly on the shoe

2. CUFF BREAK

THE RISE AND FALL OF PANTS

RISE Measures from the crotch to the top of the waistband. Measurements normally reflect a person's height (short, regular, long).
INSEAM Measures from the bottom of the crotch to the bottom of the cuff.
OUTSEAM Measures from the top of the waistband to the bottom of the cuff.
DROP The difference between the chest and waist measurements.

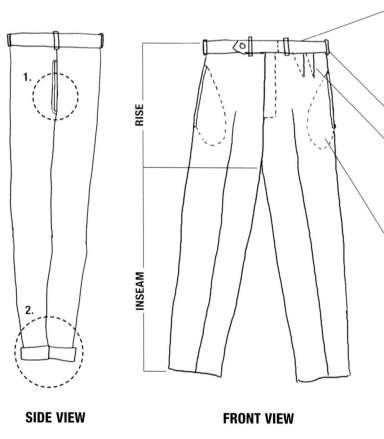

SIDE VIEW

FRONT VIEW

WAISTBAND. On casual trousers they are softer, less constructed, and can either be non-roll with expandable sidetabs or have hook closures.

GRIP. Fabric in the inside part of the waistband. Holds the shirt in place.

BELT LOOPS. Trousers with expand-able waists should not have belt loops.

PLEATS. Pleats can be "reverse" (folded inside) or "forward" (folded outside). Reverse pleats can create a slender appearance—unless the pants are too tight, in which case the bulging pleats can make you look heavier.

SIDE POCKETS. Continental, or western, pockets are cut nearly parallel to the waistband. More common (and less casual) on-seam pockets run along the outer seams with a vertical or diagonal cut.

WIDTH. Jeans or fashion-forward pants may be more narrow at the ankles than suit pants.

FLAT FRONT. Though generally infor-mal, flat-fronted trousers also happen to be favored for suits by traditional men's shop tailors.

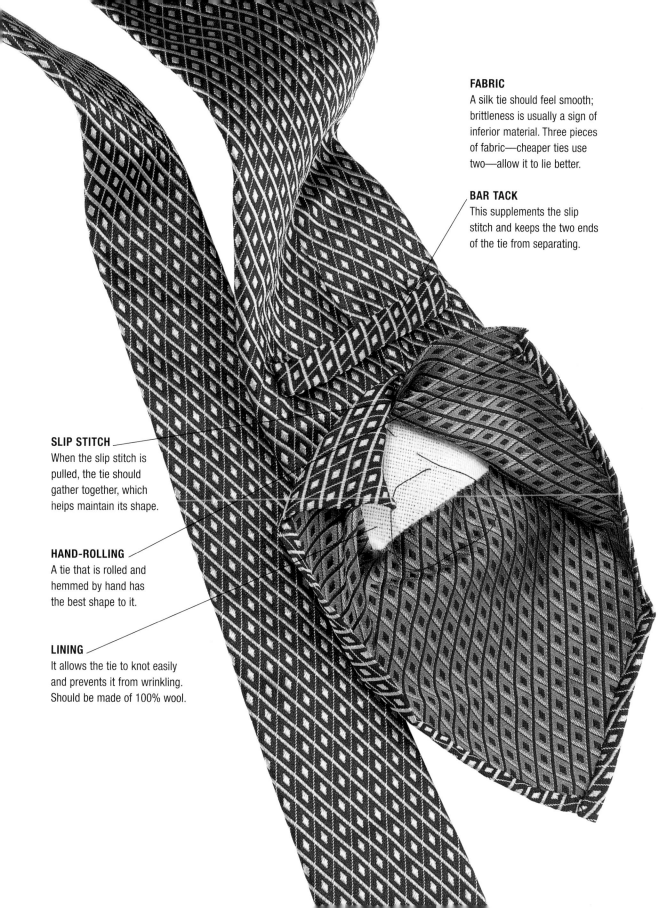

FABRIC
A silk tie should feel smooth; brittleness is usually a sign of inferior material. Three pieces of fabric—cheaper ties use two—allow it to lie better.

BAR TACK
This supplements the slip stitch and keeps the two ends of the tie from separating.

SLIP STITCH
When the slip stitch is pulled, the tie should gather together, which helps maintain its shape.

HAND-ROLLING
A tie that is rolled and hemmed by hand has the best shape to it.

LINING
It allows the tie to knot easily and prevents it from wrinkling. Should be made of 100% wool.

3. Get Better Job

Clothes Confidence
—When Dressing Is Serious Business

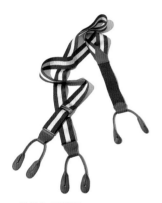

HOLD TIGHT

For the man who just can't stomach a belt and wants to try something with a little more flair, suspenders are the answer. Trousers need to have four buttons sewn into the front of the waistband and two in the back. As with ties, remember that patterns on suspenders can be very revealing. Stick with stripes and small patterns, but nothing too eccentric.

THE POWER LOOK

Now that you understand how quality connotes power, how do you actually dress to display it? One basic rule is that the more formally you are dressed, the more powerful you appear. For instance, try a blue pinstripe suit, with a white French cuff shirt and a woven silk tie. The shoes would be black cordovan cap-toes, and the belt is black alligator. Finally, just to add a splash of dash, you wear a white pocket square. The overall effect is a man in classic corporate armor who appears invulnerable.

THE POWER PALETTE

Color is another way of denoting power. In suits, dark and formidable is what you are after, so blue, gray, and black remain at the top of the power palette. White is still the most formal dress shirt, but bold patterns and colors can often signal that you have clout. Multicolored stripes and big checks are often a sign of status, as are bright pastels such as pink, orange, and green. But perhaps no color dominates the power palette these days quite like purple. As regal as it was a thousand years ago, purple has emerged in the last few years as the color to be reckoned with in a shirt and tie.

Dressing for Your Goals

IT'S NOT ALWAYS ABOUT THE CORNER OFFICE

Not everyone wants to be number one. Not everyone wants to be the biggest fish in the biggest ocean. Some don't even want to be the big piranha in the smallest lake. For these men, dressing to get ahead has a built-in ending. These are the lucky ones. They can dress for work simply to fit in, to show they are part of the club, forever. As long as they do the job, dress appropriately and respectfully, these men will go far, but not too far.

For the rest, dressing to get ahead has only been a piece—albeit a very strategic piece—of the master plan. These men want more money, more prestige. Some just want more power. Whatever your goal, it requires hard work, passion, and, yes, a closet that will work overtime for you.

PEOPLE CHANGE, GOALS CHANGE

You put in the hours, you dressed the part, and you got further than you ever expected. In fact, it's too far. You no longer have time for your friends and family. You can't catch a ball game on weekends. You're tired. All the time. This be-careful-what-you-wish-for scenario is as common as its underdog counterpart: You were ambitious from the start, but all of your effort has gone underappreciated. Is it time to get off the treadmill and realize that the dream has passed you by?

When the goals change—and almost everyone's do at least once in

3. Get Better Job

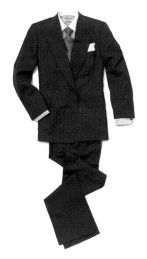

AUTHORITATIVE

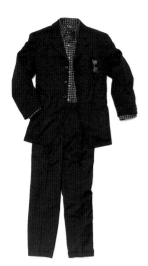

INDEPENDENT

the course of a career—it becomes necessary to reassess what is important to you. And once you do, is wearing a suit and tie really how you want to spend your days? Or, on the contrary, have you finally realized that it's time to start dressing like a grown-up? Does your image need reevaluating?

HOW TO LOOK MORE...

Professional. By now, you should know the basic tenets of looking more professional, but just to be clear, looking more professional means meeting the sartorial standards of your office or industry. No matter the standard, looking more professional most likely means going one step above where you are now: From business casual to appropriate, and from appropriate to corporate.

Trustworthy. Take a page out of the presidential candidates on this one. When they want to look like solid citizens to the rest of us solid citizens, they go with a blue suit and a white shirt and a red tie. Is it any wonder that we recommended wearing that on your first job interview? Trust us.

Authoritative. If you want to look like one of the "suits" you have to wear one. Take a look at your superiors: What do they wear? Pinstripes? Double-breasted suits? French cuff shirts? Remember, management always looks a little stiff, a little too proper, so don't overdo it.

Creative. In creative fields—such as publishing, advertising, media—dress codes are notoriously relaxed (unless your job requires that you be on camera a lot). So how do you look creative when you are supposed to be creative? Well, black usually does the trick. A black suit, a black sweater with a white T-shirt underneath, black shoes. It shows everyone that you can look professional and still maintain your personality.

Independent. Every man wants to be his own man, and looking independent is a part of that. The key is finding a way to do it without looking unprofessional. Wearing jeans to the office would not be a good approach. But always wearing a cowboy belt might be. Yes, it's a bit eccentric, but if you can stand a little criticism, soon enough it will become your trademark. Here's a range of similar ways to express independence: Bow ties, checked shirts, turtlenecks, monogrammed shirts, cowboy boots, a leather jacket. The point is, you can exert your independence in many ways—by being dandyish or rugged, bohemian or preppy—just as long as you look professional first.

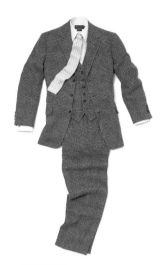

FRIENDLY

Friendly. If your image is a bit aloof, you need to warm it up. No one wants to work with someone who seems distant (what is he hiding?) or superior to them—especially if you're not. So what will make you look more friendly? You have to know your audience. If you're a white-collar guy trying to make a good impression on a blue-collar crowd, then a button-down oxford shirt and tie, with the jacket off and the sleeves rolled up, will make you seem to be a man of the people. If you appear too threatening to women, a bow tie actually declaws most men—possibly because there's almost nothing that's as asexual as a bow tie. Can you loosen up in your office? Try dressing business appropriate. Wear a sport jacket with a shirt and no tie. You will look approachable. Bright colors also work wonders. A bright tie will seem cheerful, whereas something dark can often seem funereal. Oh, and would it kill you to smile every once in a while?

Organized. If your appearance is neat and tidy—and that includes your desk and/or office—people will assume that you are organized. Even if it means sweeping all that junk into your desk, do it. No one has to know what you look like on the inside. As for clothing, it wouldn't hurt to be a little fastidious. Keep your pants creased, your shoes polished, and your shirts pressed. Your ties should always be knotted to the top. And make sure your watch is set five minutes ahead.

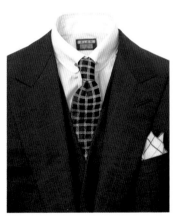

AFFLUENT

Affluent. Sad, but true, some people do judge a book by its cover. If you want to invest in two areas that can make you seem like you're packing a big portfolio, splurge on a good pair of shoes and a nice watch. The shoes you can't really skimp on—you don't need to spend $1,000 but $200 is about right—but a watch doesn't need to cost more than $100 to look expensive. These days, Timex, Swatch, Fossil, and other manufacturers put enough bells and whistles on their timepieces that you can fool almost anyone.

3. Get Better Job

Your Personal Dress Code

MONOGRAMS FOR GENTLEMEN

Whether it's a custom-made shirt or store bought, one way to assert yourself and your style is through monograms. There are only two options on where to put them: On the left chest (on the pocket or where it would be, when there isn't one) or on your sleeve cuff. Reserve it to three letters and pass on any designs. The fact that you have a monogram says enough.

DRESSING FOR YOURSELF

As you start your career there are many rules to follow—whom you should get to know, how you should behave, what you should wear—but over time, you start to make your own rules. Naturally, you still have to remain within the boundaries of professionalism and keep playing the long game, but you can (and should) find your own way sometimes. So it is with dressing. You can dress smart, dress by the book, forever, but you will never truly become your own man if you do.

PERSONAL STYLE—THE MARK OF AN INDIVIDUAL

You can purchase the perfect wardrobe over the years, but you still have to know how to put it all together. How you do that, and the way you carry yourself, will define your personal style. Are you somewhat preppy? Do you dress urban? Bohemian? Or are you still searching for your signature look?

Perhaps the simplest way to express your individuality is with shirts and ties. Nothing allows a man to stretch himself and show what he's really like as shirts and ties do. You can be bold, whimsical, somber, just about anything you'd like to be. Accessories are another way for men to show their individuality. Because we don't wear much jewelry, that basically leaves items such as cuff links, pens, belts, shoes, etc., for a man to reveal who he is.

UNIFORM DECISIONS

One of the best ways to express individuality is to wear a uniform to work. Not a real uniform, of course, not unless you're, say, a waiter or a concierge. Rather, you can develop a signature look that will come to be your personal uniform. It may be as simple as always wearing a blue suit—and having six or seven of them—every day with a blue shirt and tie, but even that kind of monotony can come to express individuality.

A uniform can also be a smart statement because once you find something that looks flattering on you, you will want to stay with it. If a three-button black suit with a white shirt looks best on you, stick with it.

A SIMPLE PALETTE

Just as wearing a professional uniform can demonstrate who you are, so, too, can having a signature color. In general, it's best to stay with basics and neutrals: navy, black, gray, tan, etc. They are safe colors—no one really looks bad in them—and everything mixes well with them. And when you're heading off on a business trip, it will reduce the packing headaches considerably.

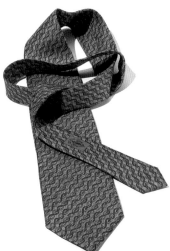

THE STATUS TIE

In the 80s, the Hermès tie signified power. Its small, playful patterns—equestrian motifs, animals, bright colors—were a symbol of French luxury. The Hermès tie is still a status symbol, of course, but now it has some company. Other luxury labels—Gucci, Chanel, and even Brooks Brothers—have all started turning out ties with similar savoir faire.

WORK EMERGENCY KIT: OFFICE

You dress carefully every day, you are a shining example of shining examples, with every tie dimpled, with every pant break just right—so why is it that the afternoon you come back from your daughter's soccer game in your less than pristine sport coat your boss calls and says she needs you to come and meet the important new client? The remedy: Keep an emergency kit in your office that allows you to do the Clark Kent.

❏ Navy-blue blazer in a year-round fabric, like high-performance wool

❏ White cotton shirt with point collar (easier to dress up for last-minute appointments than a button-down collar)

❏ Pair of solid gray worsted wool pants

❏ Sold dark tie or black knit tie

❏ Black leather belt

❏ Dark colored wool or cotton socks

❏ Black shoes: Oxfords with leather soles, or simple loafers

❏ Shaving kit and toothbrush

❏ Disposable shoe-shine wipes

Power Wardrobe

At the beginning of your career, you dressed appropriately to show respect. But at this point you want to have the respect of others, and the first step toward achieving that goal is dressing with authority. Looking the part is obviously not enough when it comes to acquiring power in the workplace—you have to earn that—but how you present yourself signals more than ever your position and prestige. By now, your seniority has also provided you with the resources to invest in the proper clothing befitting your status. This chapter will present the appropriate suits, shirts, ties, and accessories of the power wardrobe. Acquiring a power wardrobe is not simply about the amount of clothing you have—although the more options you have at this stage of your career, the better. What you're after now is quality. Finer materials and better-made clothing are what distinguish the distinguished at this level. And when you have truly achieved a certain level of power, the power wardrobe will be incidental: Your own personal style will matter most.

"The power to define the situation is the ultimate power."

JERRY RUBIN

Growing (Up) at Thirty-Seven

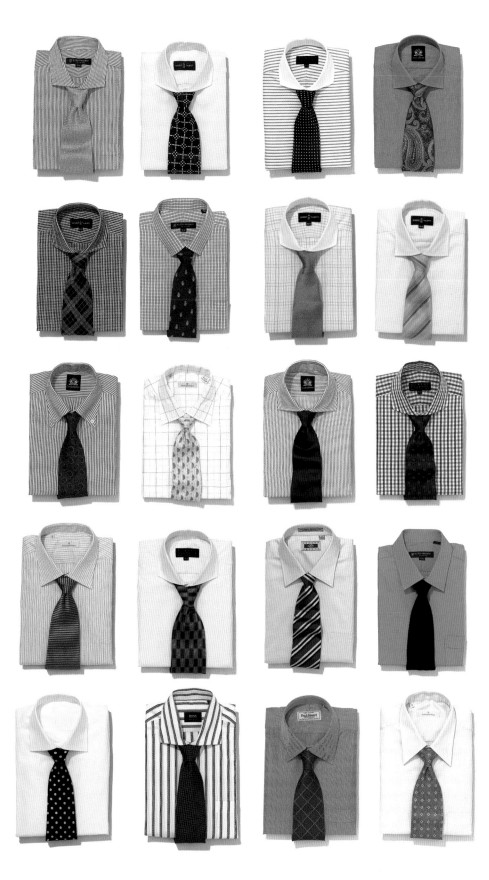

Navy
Wool Crepe

Unlike the navy suit you interviewed in, the wool crepe suit has a textured and slightly nubby feel to it. Wool crepe is more twisted than the worsted that most suits are made of, which means that it will wrinkle less. This makes a wool crepe suit ideal for travel. You can wear it on the plane or pack it without the fear of looking like a rumpled mess when you arrive. Like the original interview suit, a navy wool crepe suit goes with just about every shirt-and-tie combination. An overall bulletproof selection.

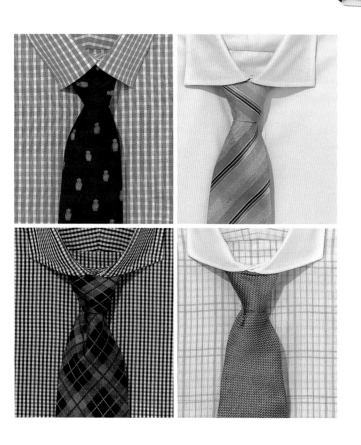

Gray Bird's-Eye

The name of the pattern refers to the minute black-and-white woven design, which actually looks gray. A smart-looking variation on the gray worsted wool suit, the bird's-eye has a lot of texture. Keep in mind that although it looks like a solid from far away, up close it is actually a very tiny pattern, so don't mix it with small-patterned shirts and ties.

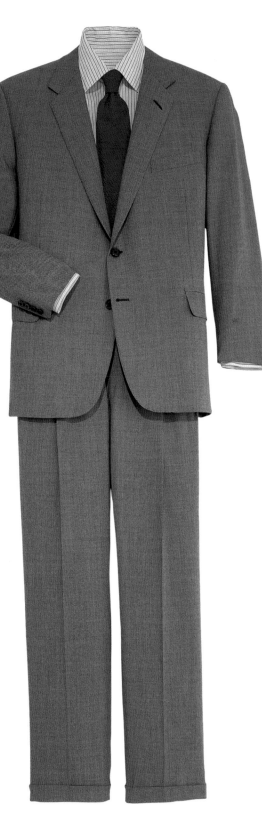

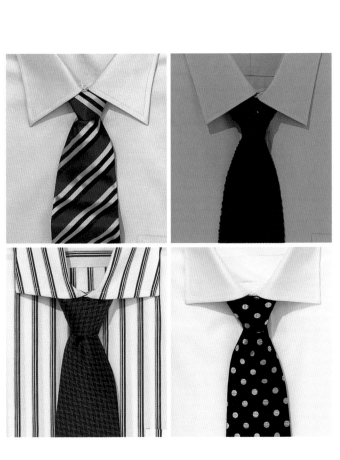

Single-Breasted Pinstripe

While not as dandyish as the double-breasted version, this suit is no less formal. What matters here is the pinstripe: It is the pattern of power. It's also the most slimming design for heavier men—the vertical stripes provide the illusion of height and diminish width. When choosing a shirt, beware of stripes that fight with the stripes of the suit. And for an added flourish, try a pocket square or a handkerchief.

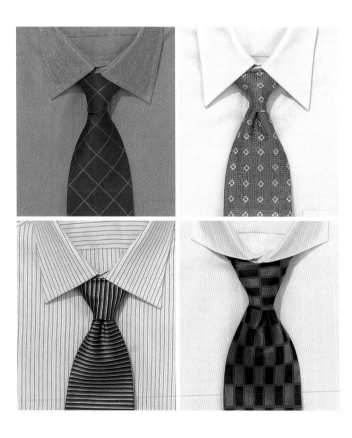

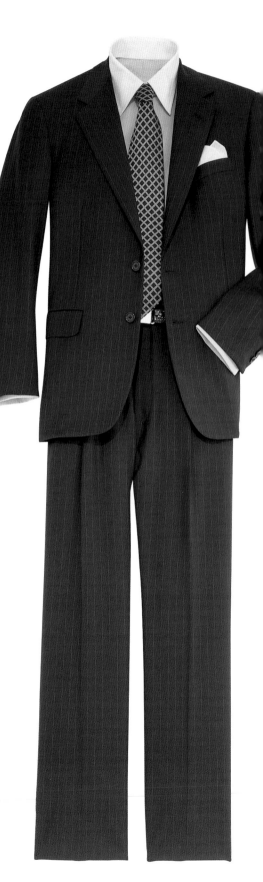

Tan Gabardine

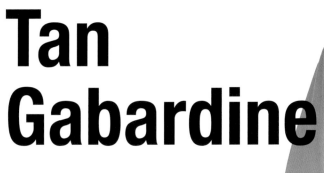

Think of it as the navy suit for warm weather. If you live in a cold-weather city, it's ideal for spring and summer; in warm locales it's appropriate all year-round. When pairing shirts and ties with this suit, remember to keep them relatively light. White or light blue shirts will always work, and pale pastels are safe as well. In terms of ties, you can go a bit darker than the shirts, but in general navy or dark green would be the safest.

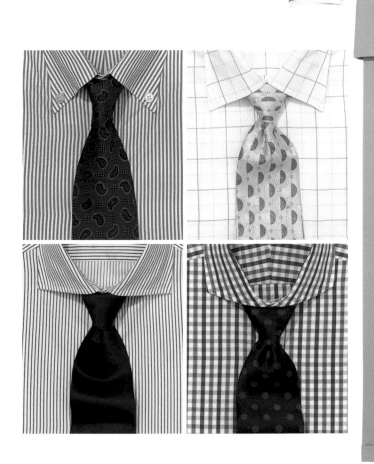

Double-Breasted Pinstripe

This classic style and pattern adds up to a suit you can take to the bank. Or a lawyer's office. Or an important business meeting. Double-breasted—meaning the left side of the jacket buttons on the right side—is a more dramatic suit cut than single-breasted, providing greater impact. (It's also the cut that all the 40s gangsters wore.) The wide lapels often scare some men away, but as long as you don't look as though an F-14 can land on your chest, you're safe. In all, this is a classic suit that defines power.

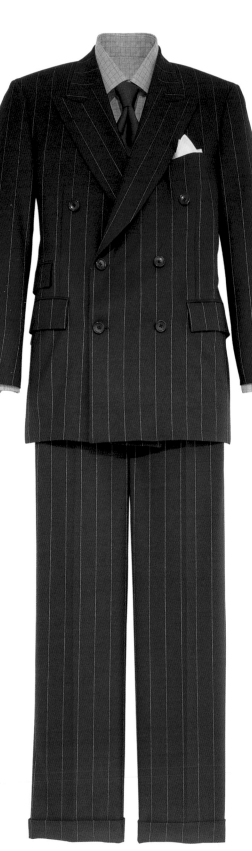

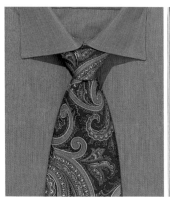
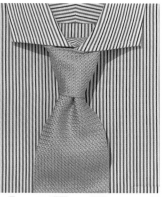
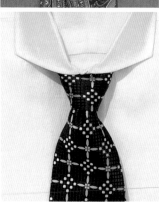
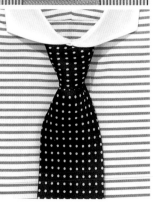

Attention to Detail

Okay, so you'll never be a designer, but you still like your clothes a certain way—shirts that are wider in the chest, collars that are spread extra wide—and now you can afford to have them tailored just for you.

MADE TO ORDER

A custom-made shirt is unquestionably an extravagance, but it's also a great way to express your sartorial individuality. Typically, from the first fitting (where a tailor will take more measurements than you knew you had) to the final product, it takes several weeks to produce a custom-made shirt. While you can expect to pay anywhere from $75 to several hundred dollars for one, the fit will be perfect. Also, the patterns and materials (frequently Sea Island or Egyptian cotton) will be superior to ready-made shirts.

SNAP COLLAR

For a more sophisticated variation on the button-down collar, try hidden snaps.

CUSTOM-MADE SHIRT

A custom-made shirt has expert stitching around the collar and placket. Look for 14 or more stitches per inch.

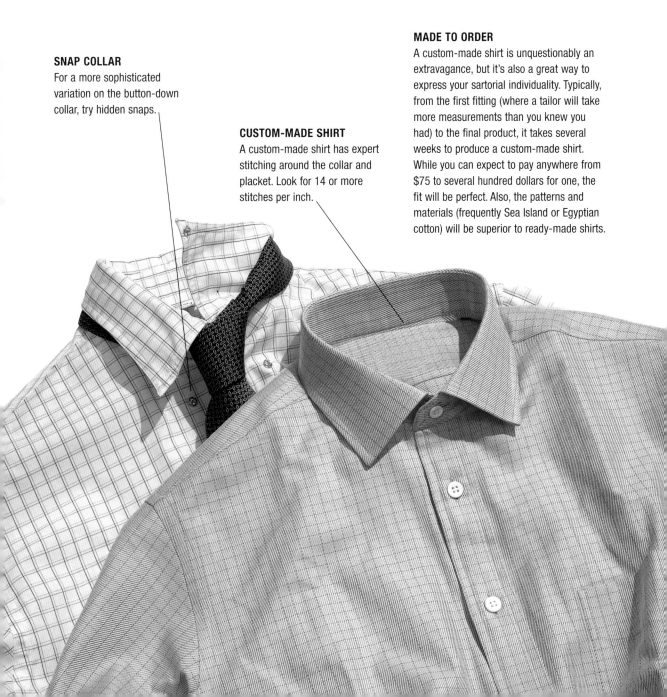

Blazers...

Like white shirts, khakis, and jeans, can a man really own enough blue blazers? Probably. But the point is, a blazer is so versatile and will get so much use that, after a while, having more than one becomes necessary. How you choose additional jackets depends on your needs: Would you like a linen blazer for summer and one in cashmere for winter? How about a double-breasted jacket instead of a single?

TWO-BUTTON
Made popular by JFK, the two-button single-breasted jacket has remained an American favorite. It flatters most, since its elongated frontal V shows more shirt, thus lengthening the line of a body.

DOUBLE-BREASTED
Traditionally, the double-breasted blazer is navy blue, with six metal buttons, only two of which actually function. Further characteristics are side vents, two flap pockets, a breast pocket, and peaked lapels. For business, metal buttons may be considered too casual. They can be replaced with horn.

THREE-BUTTON
A three-button jacket is considered fashionable. Most designers make them so only the top two buttons close, although some men prefer the more classic three, in which the lapel rolls to the second button and the top one remains unbuttoned and hidden behind the lapel.

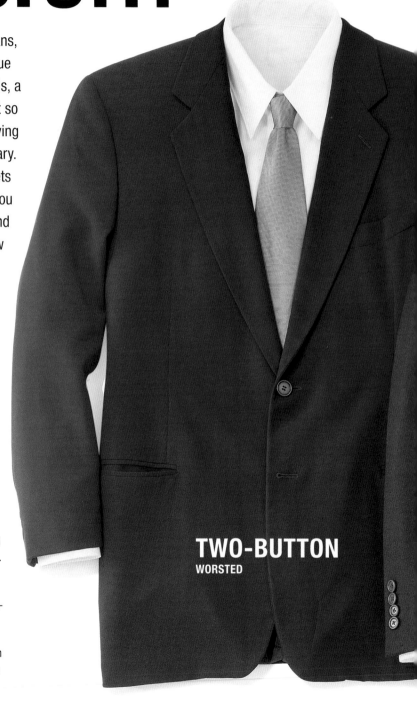

TWO-BUTTON
WORSTED

a Wardrobe of Basics

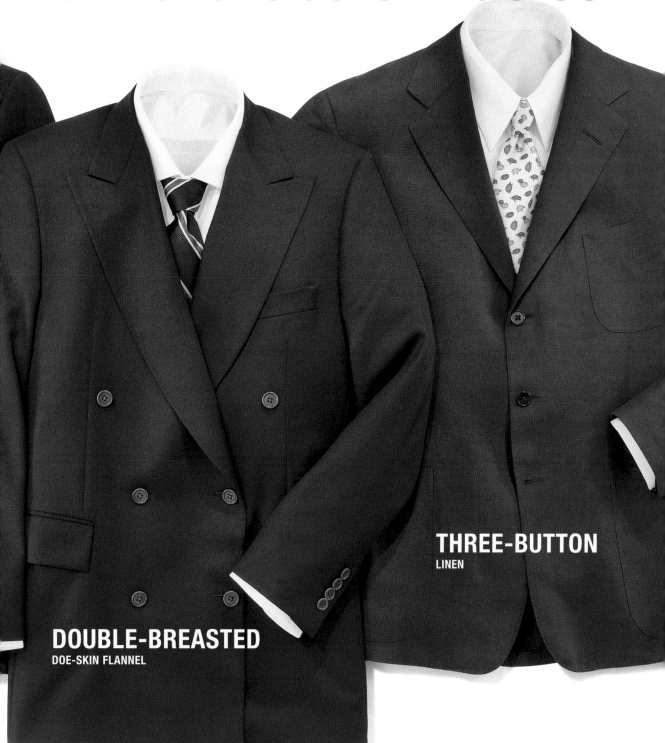

DOUBLE-BREASTED
DOE-SKIN FLANNEL

THREE-BUTTON
LINEN

Shirt & Tie Combinations

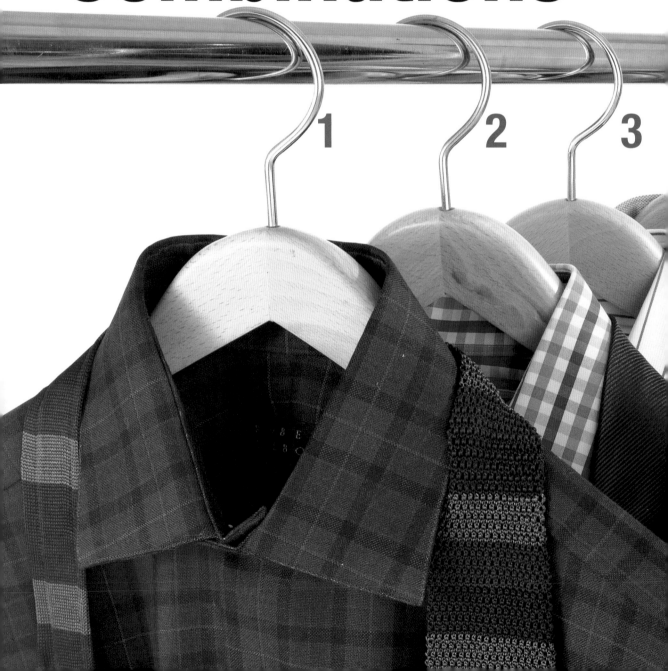

As you spend more money on shirts and ties, mixability becomes essential. Why have a $100 tie if it only goes with one shirt and suit? So, when expanding this area of the wardrobe, think about all the potential combinations with your existing clothes. Solid ties are particularly versatile, as they go with even the wildest patterned shirt (assuming, of course, that the tie picks up a color in the shirt). In general, though, you want the tie to relate to a color in the shirt or jacket. **1.** Plaid shirt with spread collar and striped knit tie. **2.** Gingham shirt with solid navy tie. **3.** Multistripe shirt with tonal tie. **4.** Lavender oxford with small pattern tie. **5.** Blue herringbone with rep tie. **6.** Multistripe with contrast collar and tonal tie **7.** Black shirt without tie.

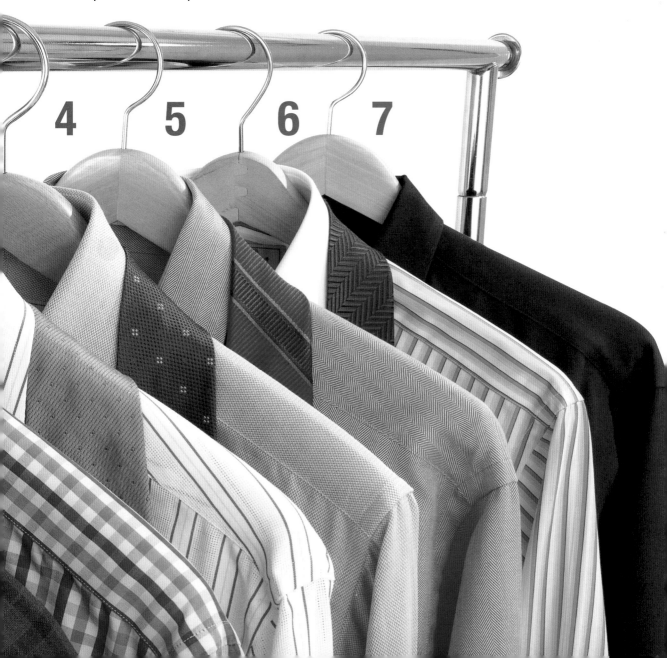

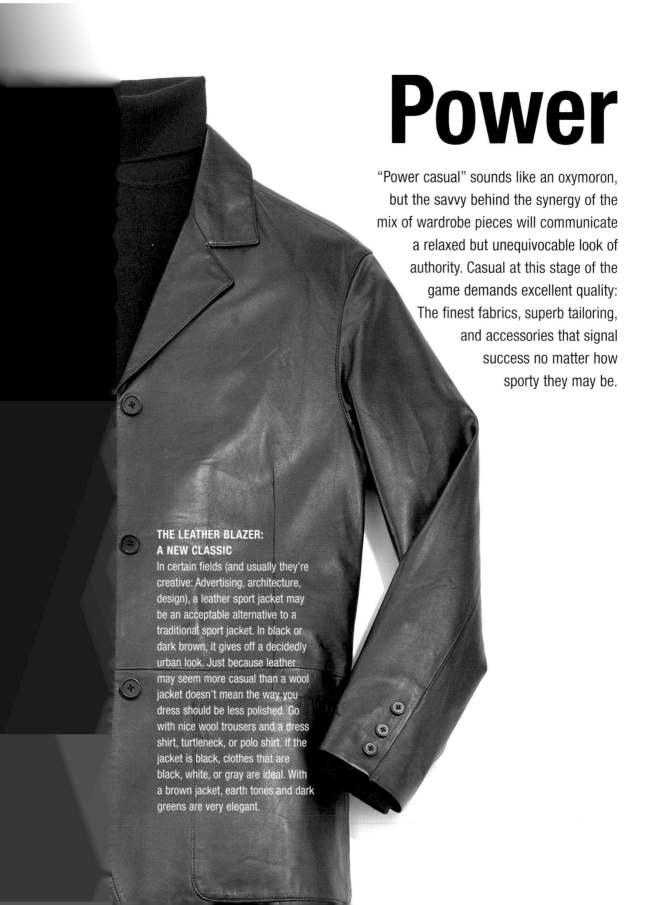

Power

"Power casual" sounds like an oxymoron, but the savvy behind the synergy of the mix of wardrobe pieces will communicate a relaxed but unequivocable look of authority. Casual at this stage of the game demands excellent quality: The finest fabrics, superb tailoring, and accessories that signal success no matter how sporty they may be.

THE LEATHER BLAZER: A NEW CLASSIC

In certain fields (and usually they're creative: Advertising, architecture, design), a leather sport jacket may be an acceptable alternative to a traditional sport jacket. In black or dark brown, it gives off a decidedly urban look. Just because leather may seem more casual than a wool jacket doesn't mean the way you dress should be less polished. Go with nice wool trousers and a dress shirt, turtleneck, or polo shirt. If the jacket is black, clothes that are black, white, or gray are ideal. With a brown jacket, earth tones and dark greens are very elegant.

Casual

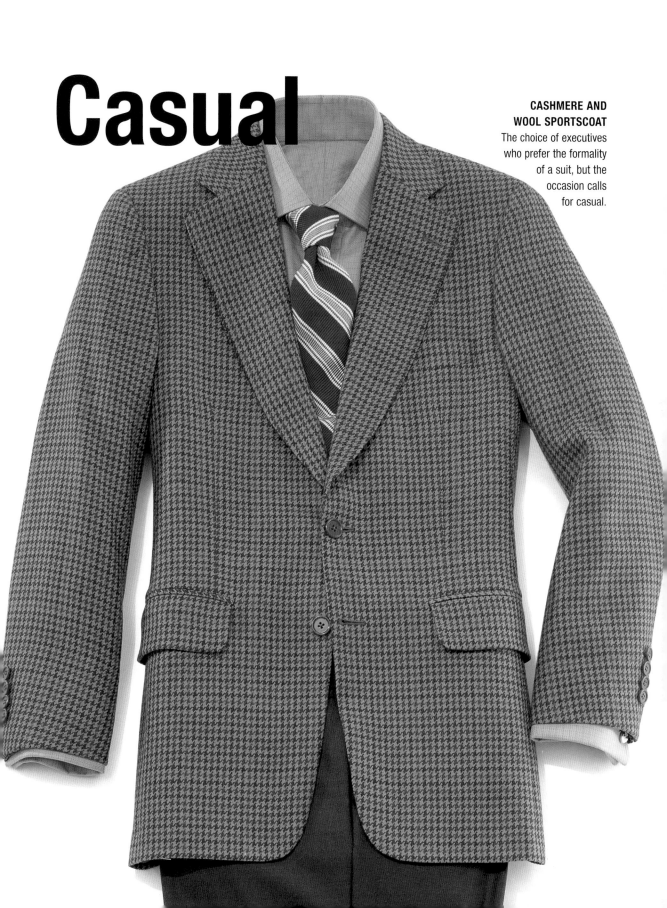

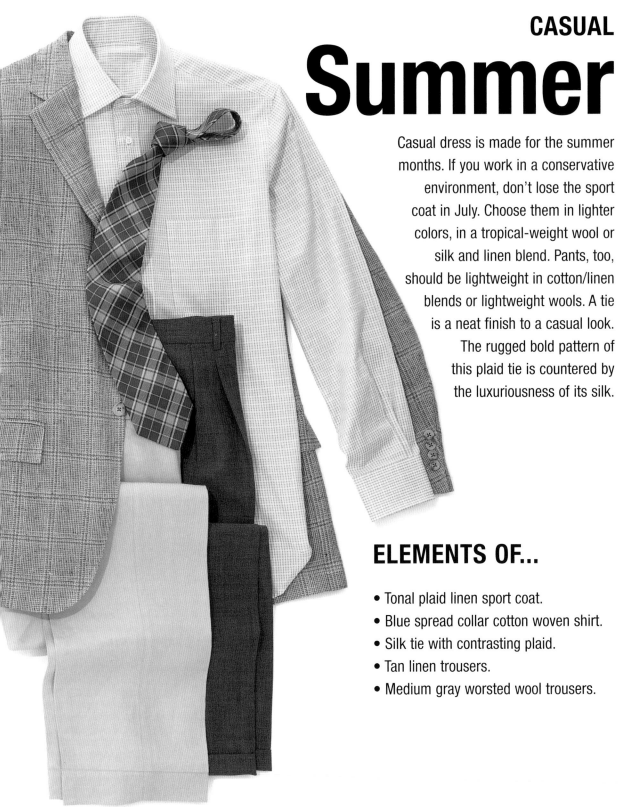

Summer

Casual dress is made for the summer months. If you work in a conservative environment, don't lose the sport coat in July. Choose them in lighter colors, in a tropical-weight wool or silk and linen blend. Pants, too, should be lightweight in cotton/linen blends or lightweight wools. A tie is a neat finish to a casual look. The rugged bold pattern of this plaid tie is countered by the luxuriousness of its silk.

ELEMENTS OF...

- Tonal plaid linen sport coat.
- Blue spread collar cotton woven shirt.
- Silk tie with contrasting plaid.
- Tan linen trousers.
- Medium gray worsted wool trousers.

CASUAL
Winter

If you are looking for luxury, cashmere is top choice, whether it's blended with wool in a sport coat, or providing that extra layer of warmth in a sweater. Super 100 wools are also a superb choice for pants and jackets and excellent for travel, as the fabric is so tightly woven it's almost impossible to wrinkle. Wide wale corduroy pants, while more sporty, are rich in texture and dress up with a sport coat and tie.

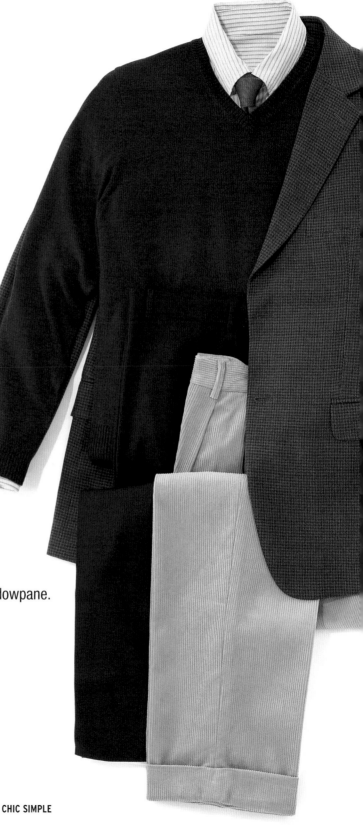

STYLE

- Tonal tweed sport coat with contrast windowpane.
- Bengal stripe button-down collar shirt.
- Contrast woven silk tie.
- Charcoal cashmere V-neck sweater.
- Charcoal flat-front worsted wool pants.
- Cream cotton corduroy pants.

Corporate

It says casual with finesse. Say it best with special details and superb fabrics—well-tailored, pleated wool pants, a rich cotton check shirt elegantly finished with French cuffs, and a sport coat with a ticket pocket and worked in Super 100 wool. Add the luxury of cashmere, which is not lost on a tie.

ELEMENTS OF...

- Tonal multiplaid wool jacket with ticket pocket.
- Tan windowpane spread-collar shirt with French cuff and silk knot.
- Cashmere tie with contrasting plaid.
- Tan worsted wool pants.
- Brown twill pants.

CASUAL
In the Field

What you wear speaks to the situation. It demonstrates that you know your territory. You have the experience. You can handle things, whether in a boardroom or in the field. If denim is appropriate, keep it dark and neat. Team it with equally substantial items: A moleskin blazer, a rich cotton tattersall shirt, a wool tie.

STYLE

- Camel moleskin sport coat.
- Broadcloth windowpane spread-collar shirt.
- Small-pattern silk tie.
- Dark denim jeans.
- Black cotton corduroy pants.

Shoes

Few things signal that a man is well-dressed like his shoes. And as the quality of your suits, shirts, and ties improves, so must your footwear. On more relaxed days in the office, loafers—either tassled or

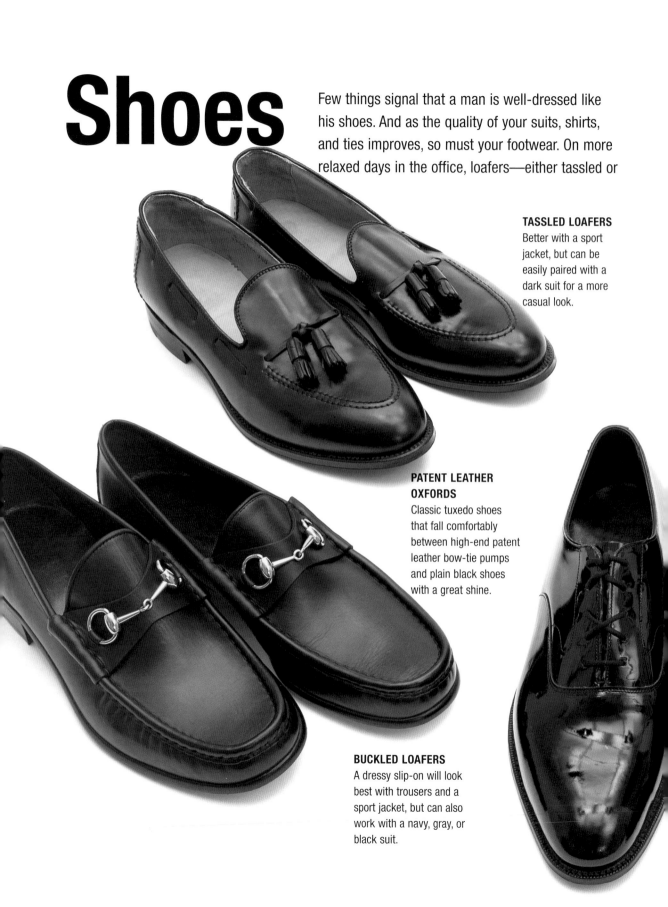

TASSLED LOAFERS
Better with a sport jacket, but can be easily paired with a dark suit for a more casual look.

PATENT LEATHER OXFORDS
Classic tuxedo shoes that fall comfortably between high-end patent leather bow-tie pumps and plain black shoes with a great shine.

BUCKLED LOAFERS
A dressy slip-on will look best with trousers and a sport jacket, but can also work with a navy, gray, or black suit.

buckled—mix well with more casual trousers, even khakis. For clothes that are brown or other earth tones, brown shoes are essential. A pair of cap-toe lace-ups—either in brown leather or cordovan—is at the dressy end of the spectrum, while a pair of chocolate brown suede shoes is a sophisticated way to dress up a pair of more casual trousers.

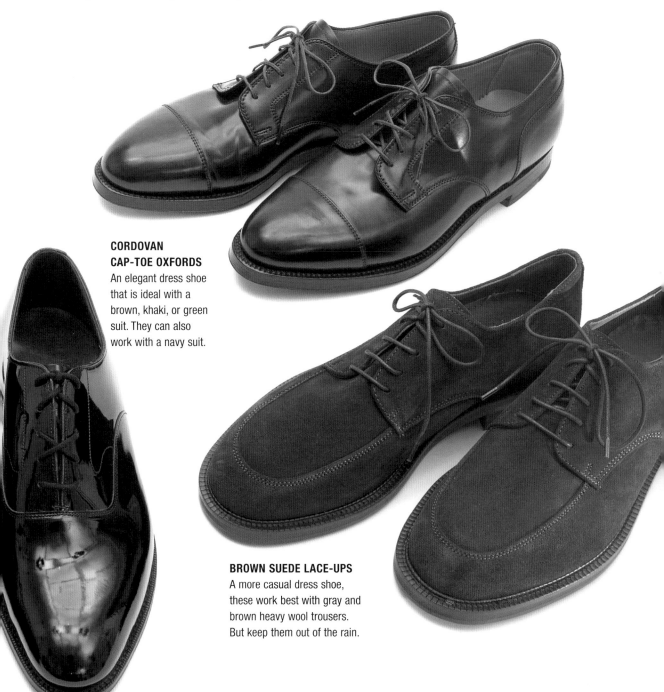

CORDOVAN CAP-TOE OXFORDS
An elegant dress shoe that is ideal with a brown, khaki, or green suit. They can also work with a navy suit.

BROWN SUEDE LACE-UPS
A more casual dress shoe, these work best with gray and brown heavy wool trousers. But keep them out of the rain.

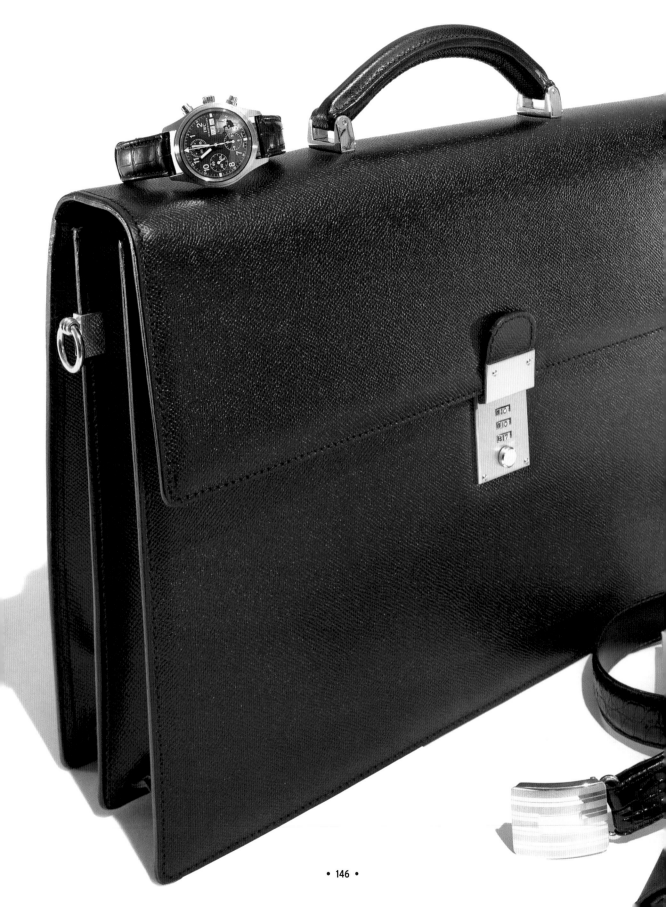

Accessories

If "God is in the details," as the architect Mies van der Rohe famously suggested, then upgrading your accessories is of divine importance. At this stage of your career, you want signature accessories, items that set you apart and display your appreciation of quality.

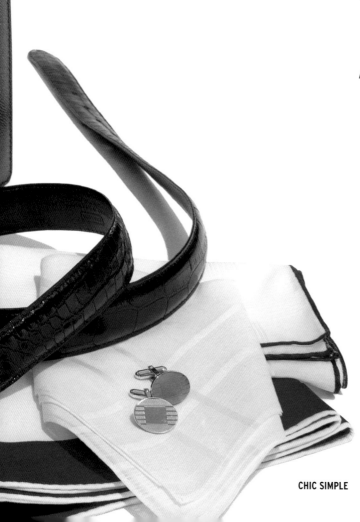

ATTACHÉ

Upgrading your leather is the first step. Improve your briefcase by choosing a more supple leather in black or brown and a more sleek, compact design. (Remember, the more powerful you are at work, the less you need to carry.) Choose a size that allows room to grow but not bulge. Look for reinforced stitching on stress points, not too many pockets (shrinks the available space), and a light-colored interior (easier to spot lost objects).

BELT WITH SILVER BUCKLE

As for your leather belts, try a skin instead (such as alligator) and perhaps a detachable silver or gold buckle that can be worn with several belts. The buckle can be engraved with your initials, but please, no nicknames.

WATCH

Your watch is the next item to upgrade; consider a sophisticated dress watch with a sporty flair, such as a pilot's watch.

CUFF LINKS

Now is also the time to build your cuff link arsenal—metals and enamels are particularly elegant.

LINEN POCKET SQUARE

Finally, though you may have been carrying a handkerchief all along, it should never be used as a pocket square. This is where the axiom "one for show and one for blow" comes in. Use a fine linen handkerchief in your jackets and save the cotton ones for your nose.

Power Coats

Upgrading your outerwear at this point typically means improving the quality of the fabric and the cut of the jacket. With overcoats, going from wool to cashmere is the way to go—it's warmer and softer to the touch.

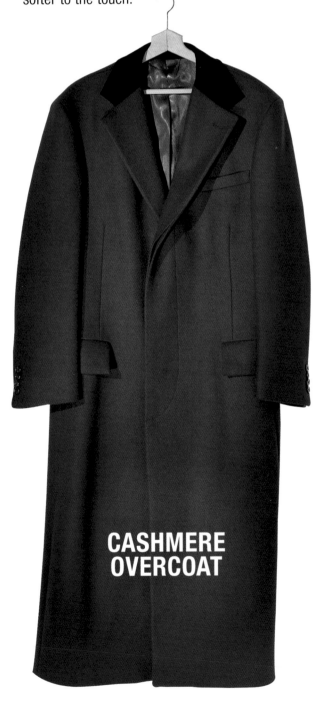

CASHMERE OVERCOAT

WHAT TO LOOK FOR

Topcoats need to cover the knee to balance the look, but they should never be so long that they drag on a long flight of steps. In black or navy, they are elegant enough to also be worn for black-tie events.

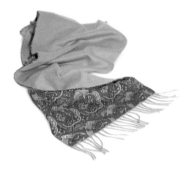

THE SILK AND CASHMERE SCARF

A silk and cashmere scarf is both practical and sophisticated, and is appropriate for all business and dress occasions.

THIN LEATHER GLOVES

A pair of thin, fine, soft leather gloves in either black, brown-black, or brown is the kind of sophisticated accessory that separates the men from the boys. Goatskin is thin and fits well; deerskin is excellent and dries without stiffening. Brown often ages into a nice mahogany, full of character and memory.

BARBOUR COAT

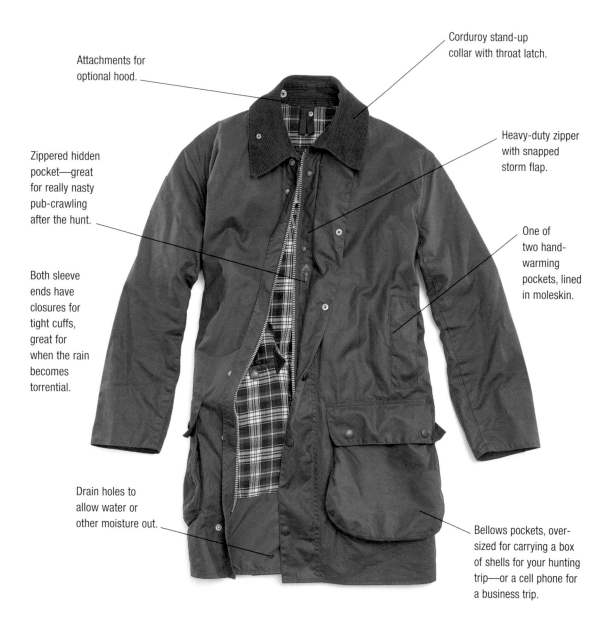

Corduroy stand-up collar with throat latch.

Attachments for optional hood.

Heavy-duty zipper with snapped storm flap.

Zippered hidden pocket—great for really nasty pub-crawling after the hunt.

One of two hand-warming pockets, lined in moleskin.

Both sleeve ends have closures for tight cuffs, great for when the rain becomes torrential.

Drain holes to allow water or other moisture out.

Bellows pockets, over-sized for carrying a box of shells for your hunting trip—or a cell phone for a business trip.

Quality outerwear not only protects you and your clothes from the elements, it also makes a statement about stature. For a rugged approach, consider some kind of hunting jacket (such as a Barbour coat) because, while it is designed to repel water and wind, it is also incredibly stylish, the very model of a British gentleman. Be sure to get a coat long enough to cover your suit jacket—you don't want the bottom hanging out.

CLOSET

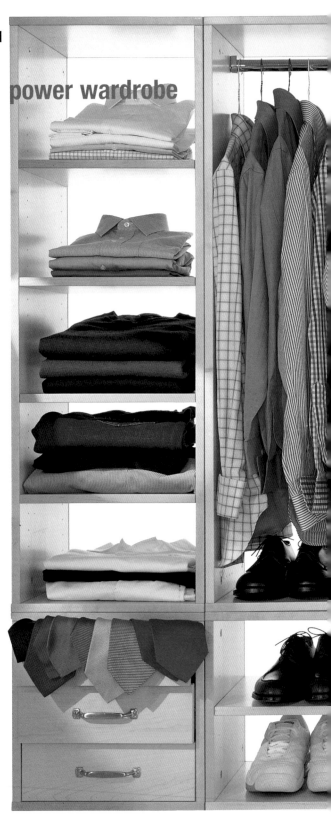

Professionally speaking, you have arrived—and settled in for a while. Your clothes shouldn't look as though they've barely survived the climb up the ladder: Your suits should be worthy of your stature. Though you may be the kind of man to give someone the shirt off your back, your shirts are far too elegant for you to do that carelessly. Your ties set you apart from other men. But does your whole closet really measure up to your place in the world? To make sure, apply the Chic Simple Process (page 19):

Assess—What do you own that is truly outdated, worn down, or simply inappropriate for this level of success?
DeJunk—Give anything away that isn't up to your standards.
ReNew—Ask yourself what's missing. A leather box to organize all your cuff links? That fountain pen you've always coveted? A second tie rack to store your neckties properly? Maybe just one more white shirt?

FEDORA TODAY

The modern-day fedora —the baseball cap— has become the headgear of choice for today's man. But with freedom comes responsibility. Here are the rules: 1. Never indoors, 2. Only when it rains or snows, 3. It should never say "I'm with stupid," 4. Should be dark in color, preferably with no logo.

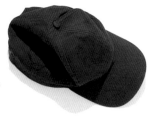

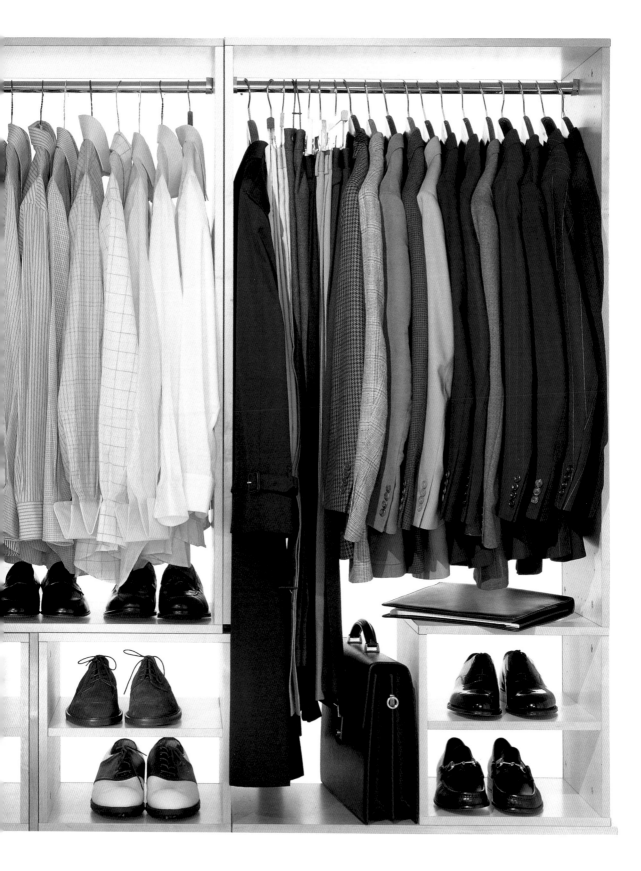

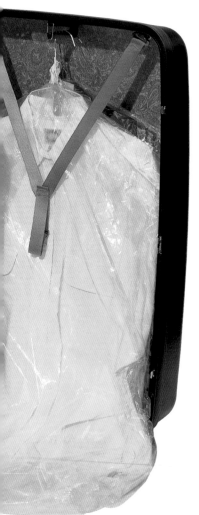

OUT OF SORTS

Dear jeff and Kim,
This is not brain surgery, but it's so annoying when my shirts and light jackets wrinkle when I travel. Garment bags, hard suitcases, and even rolling them up in a duffel—all disasters. I know I can have my shirts laundered and folded but I don't like the creases. Please don't tell me to strap them tight. I have, and that gives you a weird wrinkle across your chest. HELP!
—All Scrunched Up

Dear All Scrunched Up,
You're right, there's nothing worse than accordian pleats in your clothes and then getting them pressed for a fortune at the hotel. Have your shirts laundered and put on hangers. Ask to have each shirt in an individual piece of plastic. Hang them in your travel bag, and when you get to your destination everything looks great. What's the secret? The plastic slides against the plastic, which, like engine oil, acts as a lubricant so the cloth doesn't catch and wrinkle.

—jeff and Kim

Goes with the Job

4

Travel and Entertainment Wardrobe

What a great thing, traveling to exotic places. You get to be body searched at security and suffer the indignity of standing in your socks (with the holes in them) as you watch your shoes go through the X-ray machine. The last thing you need to worry about is the state of your wardrobe in transit. In this section we deal with not only the rigors of travel but the tightrope of letting your hair down at a business retreat while keeping your image-guard up.

Travel…
—All Dressed Up and Everywhere to Go

DRESSING FOR TRAVEL

You may be going on the road for business, but the need to dress smart is riding shotgun with you. In fact, you may have to dress even smarter. Remember, once you're out of the office, you are representing not only yourself, but also your company, so appearances matter just as much and perhaps more. What makes business travel particularly tricky for most is knowing what and how much to pack, how to make it all work together, and whether what you've selected is appropriate for where you will be. As always, preparation is the key to doing all of it well.

READY TO TAKE OFF?

Even people who love to travel usually loathe being in transit. The lines are long, the quarters are cramped, and there's always a problem with something, somewhere. And the last thing you want is to be uncomfortable. It's why dress codes for travel have completely disappeared over the years. Once, people wore suits (or at least a sport jacket) on planes. Now, it's sweat suits, T-shirts, shorts, and sneakers. And those are the people who are dressed up.

But when you're traveling for business, you can't afford to be seen in tennis warm-ups. Often, you are traveling with colleagues, but even if you are not, you will invariably run into one, so you have to look professional at all times.

> "I've
> never
> been there
> but my
> baggage
> goes
> there."
>
> **CAROL CHANNING**

COMFORTABLE VS. PROFESSIONAL

How you dress for travel depends on how you're traveling. Going alone by car? Dress as casually as you'd like, unless you have a meeting to attend as soon as you arrive. Traveling by train? A suit won't get too wrinkled over a few hours. If flying somewhere, it's best to wear your heaviest clothes and pack your lightest. A suit can get pretty roughed up by a heavy shoulder bag and general airport dirt, so go with a blazer and trousers if you can. And remember, always dress for arrival, not departure.

LOST LUGGAGE BLUES

One of the best reasons to look professional on a plane trip is that luggage has an uncanny knack for getting lost. If that tragedy should befall you, at least you will be dressed in business appropriate and can improvise for the rest of your stay. It's always wise to hedge against luggage being lost by packing toiletries in a carry-on. (Important medicine should always be carried on.) If you're going to a warm weather destination—say, for a sales conference—add a T-shirt and bathing suit to the carry-on essentials. Worst case scenario, you can sweat it out on the beach while the airline finds your bag.

location, location, location
REGIONAL AND INTERNATIONAL GUIDELINES

Politics may still be local, but dress codes no longer are. If you look professional, the specific dress codes for a region don't matter as much, but they can give you the competitive edge if you take local styles and climate into account. Here are some basic guidelines.

Think Global, Dress Local

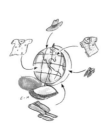

MIDWEST (CHICAGO, DETROIT, ST. LOUIS)

In the urban areas of the Midwest, the corporate and business appropriate dress codes apply: Men wear suits and ties or sport jackets and nice trousers.

NORTHEAST (BOSTON)

With all those universities, Boston can be a bit tweedy, but for business, stay with corporate and business appropriate.

NORTHEAST (NEW YORK)

New York City is the fashion capital of America, which means that just about anything goes—as long as you look good. On Wall Street and in law firms, suits (and/or jackets) and ties still reign supreme, but in the more creative fields (publishing, journalism, advertising) you need to show your personality more. A suit with a T-shirt? Turtlenecks in the office? All black? But of course. Black can be a uniform for some but not everyone can pull it off without looking like a member of a high school stage crew. If in doubt, throw in some color— say, white or gray.

MID-ATLANTIC (PHILADELPHIA, BALTIMORE, WASHINGTON, DC)

Suits are more required in Washington than in Baltimore and Philadelphia, but in any of these cities, business appropriate would be as casual as you would want to get.

PACIFIC NORTHWEST (SEATTLE)

Comfort is king here. Yes, you will find men in suits or in a jacket and tie, but business appropriate and business casual are perfectly acceptable here. And don't forget to bring a good foul-weather jacket and umbrella to combat all that rain.

WEST COAST (LOS ANGELES)

In LA, if you don't work in the entertainment industry, you wouldn't make a sound if you fell. At least that's the way you may feel. Financial executives typically wear a dark suit and tie or a suit without a tie—and of course a cell phone and car are mandatory. More creative executives also wear suits, but they are usually dressed much hipper (this season's designer labels) and more laid-back (an Armani suit with a simple white shirt). Even if an executive doesn't wear a suit, it's business appropriate all the way—with designer labels. If you're a movie star, wear whatever the hell you want.

WEST COAST (SAN FRANCISCO)

San Francisco is a cosmopolitan city and men are seen in suits or business appropriate dress. Remember, although San Francisco is in California, its climate is much cooler, so be prepared with a coat in August.

THE ROCKIES (DENVER)

Business casual with a western twist is appropriate for work in the Rockies: Khakis and a shirt with a sweater, and a good pair of boots. A sport jacket is optional, and could be worn at night.

SOUTHEAST (ATLANTA)

Atlanta is conservative, but the temperatures can get so oppressive that you may be tempted to ditch the tie. Don't. Instead, bring your lightweight suits—tropical wools, linens, poplins—and wear light colors.

SOUTHWEST (TEXAS)

Lightweight suits with ties or business appropriate clothes in light colors are the smart way to beat the Texas heat. And unless you have an authentic, serious pair of cowboy boots, just walk away from that look, hoss. And that goes double for a cowboy hat.

TROPICAL (FLORIDA)

Business attire in Florida is tropical, but not casual. Business appropriate is preferred for a meeting, but look sharp. Lightweight fabrics and light colors (even pastels) work well in Florida.

Dress Smart All Over the World

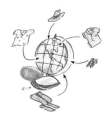

AFRICA

Dressing neatly and cleanly is respectful. English-speaking countries are more formal, less so in French-speaking countries. Avoid safari clothes for business; they can be seen as an offensive reminder of colonialism. Above all, stay away from camouflage or military dress—you could be perceived as a mercenary.

ASIA

Hong Kong: China is a very conservative country. Look corporate and wear lightweight fabrics.

Japan: Formal businesswear is the rule—wear dark suits and serious ties. Also, learn the rules of bowing; this is a crucial element of Japanese business. The exchange of business cards is almost ceremonial. The proper way is to present your card held in two hands with the print facing the recipient. When you are the recipient, receive the card with care and respect. Take a few moments to read the business card you have been given before tucking it carefully away. Do not write on a business card. It would be considered insulting. Also avoid direct eye contact.

Philippines: Among the most dapper dressers in Asia, Filipinos expect formal business attire.

EUROPE

Business dress throughout Europe is on par with dress codes in the U.S.

RUSSIA

Business attire in Russia runs the gamut from corporate to flamboyant. It is not unusual for both genders to wear an outfit several days running. Since temperatures swing to extremes, dressing in layers is advisable.

SOUTH AMERICA

Corporate business attire is customary.

AUSTRALIA AND NEW ZEALAND

Conservative work clothes are the norm. Keep in mind that the seasons are a mirror image of the North, so in December it's summer and in July it's winter.

Travel Wardrobe

Dressing for the office is often difficult enough, but choosing clothes for a business trip can be downright traumatic for some. It doesn't have to be. With proper planning and a little rigor, paring down your wardrobe for travel can be an important lesson for getting dressed in general: Learning that less is more. This chapter will discuss: 1. The smartest travel looks, 2. What to wear in transit, 3. What to pack for trips of varying lengths, and 4. The clothes and accessories that can make packing and travel easier.

"Eighty percent of success is showing up."

WOODY ALLEN

WHAT'S MY GETAWAY GEAR?

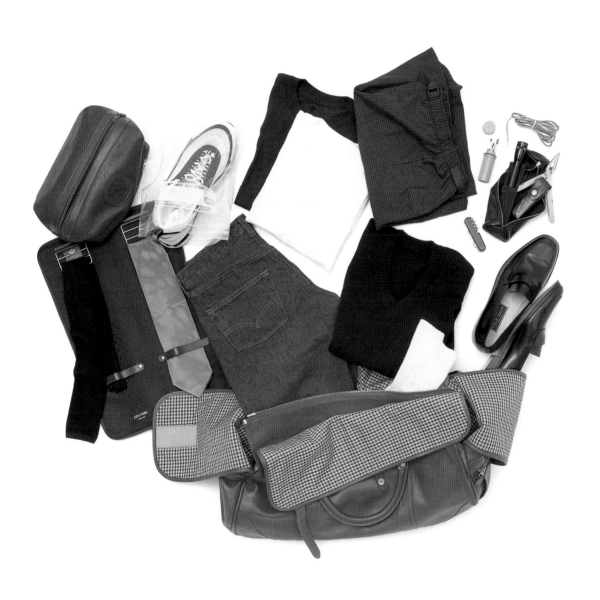

Luggage

When traveling for business, the luggage you choose must be: 1. As efficient as your filing system, 2. As presentable as your nicest suits, and 3. Practical enough to transport those suits (and shirts and shoes) to your final destination neatly and safely.

GARMENT BAG
The idea behind garment bags is that your clothing hangs in the bag exactly as in your closet. To avoid wrinkling, double-bag each garment with dry-cleaner bags.

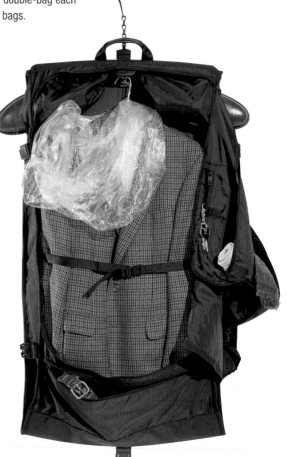

OVERNIGHTER
Your carry-on should look as respectable as you do. Be sure it's not too heavy or awkward to carry.

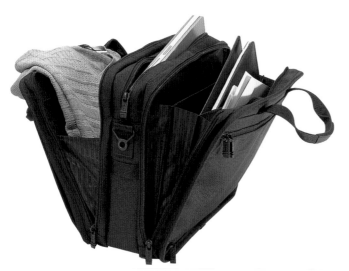

Guidelines

A WEEK OUT

Choose a style with a built-in garment bag, easy-maneuver wheels and a retractable handle that is long enough to pull without strain.

CHOOSING LUGGAGE

1. Luggage appearance is as important as your suit appearance: Pieces should match. Dark, solid colors are preferable, and make sure there are no tears or holes.
2. There's no shame in using luggage with wheels. It's easier to maneuver and won't leave you all sweaty from hauling your suitcases through an airport.
3. Bags should always have proper ID (such as a business card), and should have a colorful tag to make them easier to spot.
4. Place a copy of your itinerary in the suitcase for easy contact in case it is lost.
5. Carrying a duffel bag on a business trip is like wearing sweatpants to a board meeting.
6. Select a hanging bag that allows you to use your own hangers.
7. Your luggage will get beaten up, so choose a sturdy fabric such as ballistic nylon. It is one of the strongest at about 1,000 denier (a number system indicating width and strength of the fibers). For the average business traveler, about 420-denier nylon or 600-denier polyester should be adequate.

TRAVEL KITS

Travel kits are to travel what medicine cabinets are to bathrooms. They should be durable and spill-proof. Insist on a wide mouth with a strong zip closure and at least one interior pocket. Keep your toiletries packed for quick getaways.

DOPP STORY

Men's travel kits are often referred to as Dopp Kits. The term comes from a Chicago leather goods manufacturer called Dopp, who successfully marketed the bags.

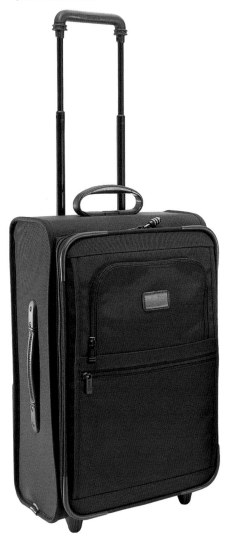

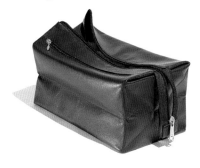

What to Pack

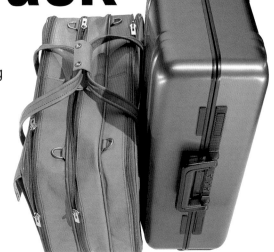

There are some foolproof methods for packing wisely and efficiently for a business trip. Employing them will prepare you for every potential hazard along the way, and relieve some of the inevitable stress that travel can cause.

ASSESS: Your travel plans. Where are you going? For how long? With whom will you be meeting? What are the weather conditions?
CONSIDER: Dress codes. What is the purpose of your trip? Is it a conference set at a resort or a meeting with potential clients? What country or region of the country are you visiting, and how do they dress there? What types of situations will you likely find yourself in—meetings, dinners, presentations? What are you most comfortable wearing?
PLAN AHEAD: Does the hotel have fax machines, computer connections, etc.? Is there a dry-cleaning service? A gym?

TEN RULES OF SMART PACKING

1. Make a checklist of what you'll need.

2. Pack as little and as lightly as possible.

3. Shoes can carry socks, belts, and small personal items (travel clock, etc).

4. Wear your heaviest shoes for traveling.

5. Empty your pockets before packing clothes.

6. Have dress shirts professionally cleaned and folded—they pack smaller.

7. Use travel-size toiletry products.

8. Place anything that might leak (lotion, suntan oil, shampoo) in a Ziploc bag.

9. Bring extra Ziplocs—great for sweaty gym clothes, wet bathing suits…

10. Always bring a pair of wool socks for cold feet in air-conditioned rooms.

...One Week

The power of a packing chart is that it eliminates the paranoia of forgetting key items, i.e. the swimsuit for the resort, gym clothes, or your black socks. To determine the minimum amount of clothes needed for the maximum amount of activities on a given trip, a packing chart can serve as an effective visual aid. Don't be anal, just fill it in based on what you need.

DAY	A.M.	P.M.	EXTRAS
MONDAY - TRAVEL DAY	navy suit	ditto	black loafers
TUESDAY	meeting: gray suit	navy jacket/gray pants, sweater	day: brown shoes night: black shoes
WEDNESDAY	FREE DAY!: khakis & blue sweater, SWIM STUFF	dinner meeting: gray suit (no tie)	black shoes
THURSDAY	breakfast/lunch meeting: black turtleneck w/ gray suit pants	room service!!!	black shoes
FRIDAY	SWIM, golf!	dinner meeting: navy suit, no tie	brown shoes
SATURDAY	all day conference: khakis & sweater	ditto	black shoes
SUNDAY - TRAVEL DAY	navy suit jacket, khakis	ditto	black shoes (loafers?)

The packing chart: The days you will be traveling go in a vertical column. Make three adjacent columns to designate what to wear in the A.M. and P.M. and a column for extras. Fill in what you plan to wear. Mix up clothing separates to avoid packing a lot.

How to Pack a...

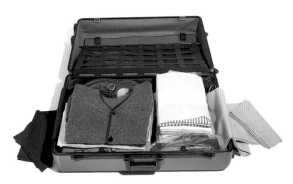

SUITCASE

1. Interlock belts and run them along the inner circumference of your suitcase.
2. Pack heavy or bulky items—shoes, toiletry kit (keep a toothbrush in your briefcase).
3. Add a layer of tissue or plastic between garments—allows clothes to slide, not rub, preventing wrinkling.
4. To pack pants: Fold at the crease and drape lengthwise in suitcase, with legs hanging over one end. Add a layer of tissue or plastic, and leave hanging while you…
5. Add sweaters, shirts, then lighter items, and another layer of tissue.
6. Fold pant legs back across suitcase.
7. Double-bag hanging garments with plastic.
8. Bring a stuff sack for other loose garments.

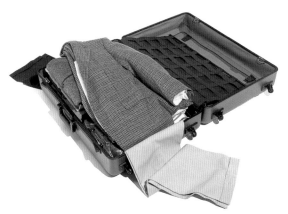

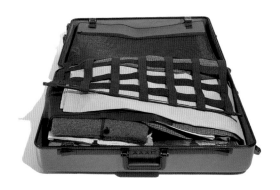

PAIR OF PANTS

1. Make sure that all pockets are empty: Keys or change may damage fabric once pants are packed. 2. Pants should be the first item packed. Place onto the bottom of bag with waistband in middle of the case, legs actually falling outside the bag. (If you are packing two pairs, place them waistband to waistband, with the legs running in opposite directions.) 3. Pack the rest of your things on top and wrap the pant legs over the pile, placing one last item over the legs to hold everything in place.

JACKET

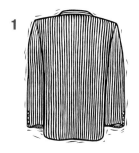 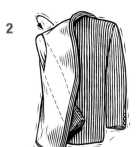 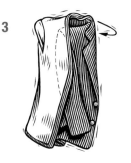 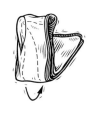

1. Empty pockets. Holding the jacket facing you, put your hands inside the shoulders.

2. Turn the left shoulder (but not the sleeve) inside out.

3. Place the right shoulder inside the left. The lining is now facing out and the sleeves are inside the fold.

4. Fold the jacket in half, put it inside a plastic bag, and place it in your suitcase.

SHIRT

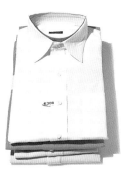

1. Button all buttons, noting which button falls below your waist.

2. Lay shirt face-down on a flat surface and fold the sleeves back at the shoulder seam.

3. Fold tail up from point of the button that is below your waistline. This will prevent shirt from having a crease across your stomach.

Note: If you can plan ahead, have your shirts cleaned and folded at the laundry before your trip.

TIE

1. Fold the tie in half. Place it on a sheet of tissue paper or length of plastic.

2. Roll it up and put a loose rubber band around the coil.

3. Place the rolled tie in the pocket of a jacket if you like before your trip.

4. Or put your ties in a tie case.

PAIR OF SHOES

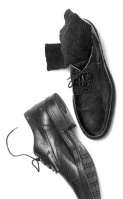

1. Shoes should always go in a bag—either cloth ones that can be cleaned, or disposable plastic bags from the grocery store.

2. Place along the edge of a hard case to keep your folded clothes from shifting.

2a. In a duffel, shoes get packed first, at the bottom.

3. Shoes can also carry socks, a coiled belt, extra eyeglasses, or overflow from your Dopp Kit, like a tube of sunscreen.

Your Travel Wardrobe

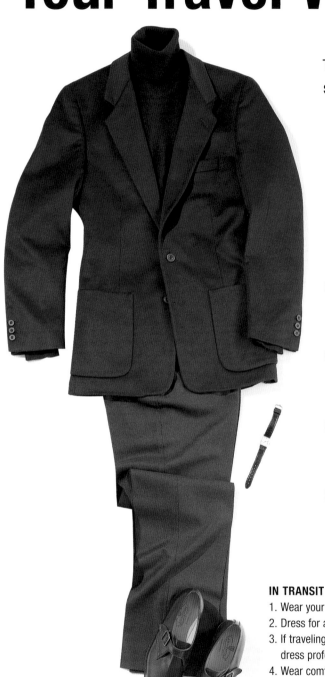

To get the most out of your wardrobe for a short road trip, consider which items work best together. A well-edited suitcase will simplify business travel and still keep you looking professional. Choose seasonless, nonwrinkle fabrics (such as lightweight wools or wool crepes). Wear mainly navy, gray, and neutrals for greater versatility.

BELT

SOCKS

BLACK KNIT TIE

LOAFERS

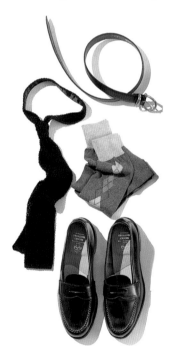

IN TRANSIT
1. Wear your heaviest clothing and shoes in transit.
2. Dress for arrival, not departure.
3. If traveling with colleagues (or going immediately to a meeting), dress professionally.
4. Wear comfortable clothes, and dress in layers if necessary.
5. A suit jacket or sport jacket is like an extra carry-on bag—it can hold tickets, a passport, glasses, pens, a phone, and a PDA.

1 navy suit + 1 blazer and slacks + 1 pair of khakis
=
6 outfits that can fit into one hanging bag.

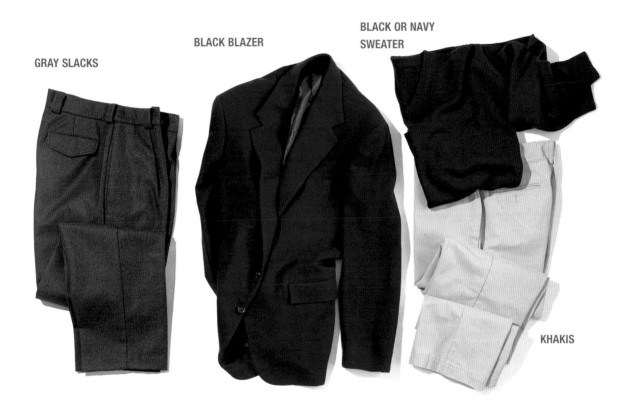

GRAY SLACKS

BLACK BLAZER

BLACK OR NAVY SWEATER

KHAKIS

GOAL
To pack your suitcase with clothes that can multitask: Key elements that can work overtime for you.

THE NAVY SUIT AND THE BLACK BLAZER
TRAVEL ASSET: These two items can be worn day or night and can be broken up into several outfits.

KHAKI PANTS
TRAVEL ASSET: A pair of khakis is excellent for traveling in—they're lightweight, comfortable, and hide wrinkles.

DAY ONE	DAY TWO	DAY THREE	DAY FOUR	DAY FIVE	DAY SIX
Black blazer	Navy suit	Suit jacket	Black blazer	Black sweater	Black blazer
Gray slacks	Shirt and tie	Khakis	Suit slacks	Gray slacks	Black sweater
Shirt and tie	Black shoes	Shirt	Turtleneck	Black shoes	Khakis
Black shoes		Black shoes	Black shoes		Black shoes

Packing Chart

ITEM	MONDAY	TUESDAY	WEDNESDAY	THURSDAY	FRIDAY	ITEM
UNDERWEAR						**UNDERWEAR**
boxers/briefs						boxers/briefs
undershirts						undershirts
HOSIERY						**HOSIERY**
socks						socks
SUIT						**SUIT**
jacket						jacket
pants						pants
SEPARATES						**SEPARATES**
sport jackets						sport jackets
pants						pants
shirts						shirts
ties						ties
ACCESSORIES						**ACCESSORIES**
briefcase						briefcase
watch						watch
glasses						glasses
sunglasses						sunglasses
SHOES						**SHOES**
lace-ups						lace-ups
loafers						loafers
sneakers						sneakers
OUTERWEAR						**OUTERWEAR**
raincoat						raincoat
coat						coat
scarf						scarf
gloves						gloves
hat						hat
umbrella						umbrella
OTHER						**OTHER**
workout						workout
swimsuit						swimsuit
evening						evening
sport						sport

REASONS FOR MAKING A PACKING LIST

1. To simplify and organize the packing process.
2. To control the number of items packed.
3. To prevent the omission of vital items.
4. To guard against overpacking.
5. To help clarify clothing options and combinations.
6. To assist with claims against lost luggage.

DAY TRIP
❏ Address book
❏ Briefcase
❏ Driver's license, identification
❏ Eyeglasses—regular, sun
❏ Handkerchief
❏ Itinerary confirmation
❏ Keys—car, home, office
❏ Medicines
❏ Money items
❏ Pens, pencils
❏ Reading materials
❏ Tickets

PACKING A WALLET
❏ Auto club membership card
❏ Billfold
❏ Business cards
❏ Cash
❏ Checkbook
❏ Credit cards
❏ Driver's license
❏ Family pictures/photographs

- ❏ Health insurance card
- ❏ Telephone card
- ❏ Traveler's checks

BUSINESS TRIP
- ❏ Address book
- ❏ Advertising materials
- ❏ Airline tickets
- ❏ Appointment book
- ❏ Briefcase
- ❏ Business cards
- ❏ Calculator
- ❏ Computer, accessories
- ❏ Confirmations—hotel, etc.
- ❏ Correspondence
- ❏ Credit cards
- ❏ Expense forms
- ❏ Files
- ❏ Highlighters
- ❏ Letters of credit
- ❏ Markers
- ❏ Meeting materials
- ❏ Money
- ❏ Notebooks
- ❏ Paper clips
- ❏ Passport
- ❏ Pens, pencils
- ❏ Portfolio
- ❏ Presentation materials
- ❏ Price lists
- ❏ Proposals
- ❏ Publications
- ❏ Purchase order forms
- ❏ Reports
- ❏ Rubber bands
- ❏ Samples
- ❏ Stamps
- ❏ Stapler, staples
- ❏ Stationery, envelopes
- ❏ Tape recorder, tapes
- ❏ Time records

A DAILY COMMUTE
- ❏ Auto club membership
- ❏ Cell phone
- ❏ Coins, tokens
- ❏ Driver's license
- ❏ Driving shoes
- ❏ Eyeglasses—regular, sun
- ❏ First aid kit
- ❏ Gas credit cards
- ❏ Keys
- ❏ Maps
- ❏ Music
- ❏ Notepad
- ❏ Pen, pencils
- ❏ Water

OVERNIGHT
- ❏ Dopp Kit
- ❏ Nightclothes
- ❏ Shirt
- ❏ Socks
- ❏ Underwear

CARRY-ON
- ❏ Address book
- ❏ Camera and film
- ❏ Confirmations
- ❏ Electronic equipment
- ❏ Eyeglasses—regular, sun
- ❏ Identification
- ❏ Keys—car, house
- ❏ Medicine
- ❏ Money
- ❏ Outerwear
- ❏ Passport, visas
- ❏ Portable CD player
- ❏ Reading material
- ❏ Ticket
- ❏ Toothbrush, toothpaste
- ❏ Water

BASIC CLOTHES
- ❏ Athletic shoes
- ❏ Belt
- ❏ Black or brown shoes
- ❏ Business suit
- ❏ Dress shirts (two white, three solid colors)
- ❏ Jeans
- ❏ Khaki or corduroy pants
- ❏ Navy blazer
- ❏ Sleepwear
- ❏ Socks and underwear
- ❏ Sports clothes
- ❏ Swimsuit
- ❏ Trench coat
- ❏ Watch
- ❏ White T-shirt

TRAVEL KIT
- ❏ Adapter kit
- ❏ Aftershave lotion
- ❏ Baggies for spillables
- ❏ Body lotion
- ❏ Cleanser
- ❏ Cologne
- ❏ Condoms
- ❏ Cotton sticks
- ❏ Dental floss
- ❏ Dentures—case, cleaner
- ❏ Deodorant
- ❏ Foot powder

- ❏ Hair care
  - ❏ Coloring
  - ❏ Comb
  - ❏ Dryer
- ❏ Lip balm
- ❏ Moisturizer
- ❏ Mouthwash
- ❏ Nail clippers
- ❏ Razor, blades
- ❏ Shampoo, conditioner
- ❏ Shaving cream
- ❏ Soap
- ❏ Soap dish
- ❏ Styptic pencil
- ❏ Sunscreen
- ❏ Tissues
- ❏ Toothbrush, toothpaste
- ❏ Tweezers

MEDICINE CHECKLIST
- ❏ Antiseptic lotion
- ❏ Aspirin
- ❏ Band-Aids
- ❏ Cold remedies
- ❏ Diarrhea medication
- ❏ Emergency contacts
- ❏ Identification bracelet
- ❏ Insect repellent
- ❏ Medical information— allergies, medications, and blood type
- ❏ Moleskin for blisters
- ❏ Physician's name, address, and telephone

- ❏ Prescription medications
- ❏ Sunblock
- ❏ Thermometer
- ❏ Throat lozenges
- ❏ Vitamins

INTERNATIONAL CHECKLIST
- ❏ Addresses for correspondence
- ❏ Auto registration (if driving)
- ❏ Cash, including some in the currency of the country to which you are traveling
- ❏ Credit cards
- ❏ Emergency contacts
- ❏ Extra prescription glasses and contacts
- ❏ Insurance papers
- ❏ International driver's license
- ❏ Lightweight tote bag for purchases
- ❏ Medical information
- ❏ Passport, visas, health certificates
- ❏ Phrase book or dictionary
- ❏ Special prescriptions and medications
- ❏ Sunglasses
- ❏ Tickets and travel documents
- ❏ Travel itinerary
- ❏ Traveler's checks and personal checks

4. Goes with the Job

… & Entertainment
—Relax, It's Only Your Career

OUT OF THE OFFICE

Unlike, say, the decathlon, business comes with events that do not have obvious rules. How does one dress professionally in situations that do not seem overtly professional? Enter "The Special Occasion Wardrobe." Whether you're playing in a corporate golf tournament or attending the company Christmas party, you never stop being an employee. In situations like these, appearances count more than ever because there is greater room for error. To select clothing for any potential "off-campus" event, from a tennis outing to a public speaking appearance to a black-tie dinner, read on.

MEALING AND DEALING

Unlike women, men know how simple it is to go from day to night: We just show up. Unless a man is wearing a very light suit that might look out of place in the evening, he doesn't give a second thought to dressing differently to go out.

And yet, the idea of business meetings that take place over drinks, meals, and at other "off-site" locales can intimidate some guys. Here are some basic rules to follow and pay attention to.

BREAKFAST, LUNCH, AND DINNER

The rules of dress don't really change for men, except that the restaurant can get more casual or dressy. But dressing at meals is something of a constant. So even if breakfast is at a diner and dinner is at a four-star restaurant, you could still wear a suit and tie to either and feel appropriate. If you are uncertain of a restaurant's standards, however, simply phone ahead and ask.

Where it gets somewhat tricky is table manners. Do not underestimate how crucial these are as well. If you are unsure of your manners, learn what is proper etiquette and follow it. Put your napkin in your lap (never over your collar!). Use silverware from the outside in. Chew with your mouth closed. Say "please" and "thank you." And try not to eat all over yourself.

DRINKS

Drinks with a client, a superior, or even a colleague can often be nerve-wracking. Not because you don't know what to wear: That's easy—just wear what you wore to work. Or, if you feel underdressed or overdressed (because of the place you are going to or the people you're meeting), dress up or down accordingly.

No, what gets tricky is knowing how much to drink. The answer? Not much. One drink, two at the most, is appropriate. Anything more and you risk getting drunk, which is just another way of looking sloppy.

BLACK TIE

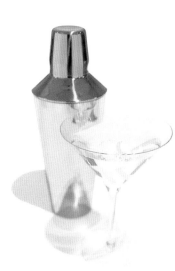

Let's be honest, wearing black tie is the greatest thing that could ever happen to a man sartorially. Put on a tuxedo and you are instantly elegant. Therefore, it's almost inconceivable that a man could mess it up, and yet it happens.

One of the most basic reasons is that most men are afraid to buy their own and so they rent: That's how you end up looking like the waiters. A tuxedo may be an expensive investment, but if you go to one or two black-tie events a year, it is well worth it. A classic tuxedo (and that's the only kind to buy) will last for five to ten years, assuming you can still fit into it.

Then, buy yourself a proper tuxedo shirt, a bow tie, some cuff links and studs, and you are set for any swank evening. Oh, and when the invitation says "Creative Black Tie"—be uncreative. Leave the flashy bow ties and black shirts to the other guys. Your attitude is this: If Cary Grant wouldn't wear it, you wouldn't wear it.

4. Goes with the Job

DANGER ZONES—DRESSING FOR "RELAXED OCCASIONS"

You know you're going to be around your colleagues for a few days, but you're out of the office. To many men, this is very complicated. Do you loosen up completely and show them what you're really like? Do you play it safe and wear the same thing you do to the office—only without a tie?

What are the rules when there are seemingly no rules?

CONVENTIONS

Attending a convention is like going to any industry event, so dress appropriately for your profession. Unlike an event that's exclusive to your company, a convention is attended by people across your industry, so now would be a good time to make a nice impression on someone outside your firm. Think of it as a job interview without all the formality.

SALES CONFERENCE

At a sales conference or corporate retreat, you are still on company time, which means you are still being watched, and perhaps judged. This is not the time to slack off. But you still want to show that you can be relaxed. In order to show that you can look professional and still wind down, dress somewhere between high business casual and low business appropriate. Khakis and dress shirts by day, throw on a blazer at night, and you can do no wrong. Jeans are fine, too, but make sure they're not ripped. Sneakers? Sure, but not if they're ragged. And if you're heading somewhere with a beach, pack a bathing suit, but remember to leave a little something to the imagination. No one is going to be impressed by seeing you in those tight swim briefs. The women in the office will wonder what you are trying to prove, and the men will just think you look foolish. Sensible trunks are the way to go.

CORPORATE ATHLETIC OUTINGS

Such clannish affairs often result in either a bonding experience or an alienating one. Clothes must be considered carefully—those you would normally wear in such a setting might send an undesirable message when you're surrounded by work colleagues. Because so much business is now conducted on the golf course, dressing smart in an athletic setting can give you the competitive edge. Golf clothes have come a long way in the last decade, and are now extremely stylish and very high-tech. There are fabrics that wick moisture away from the body, and protect against the wind and rain.

GOLF

Here are a few basic tips to make you look comfortble on the links. For starters, don't accept a golf invitation if you don't know how to play. You will only embarrass yourself. (A quick tip: Your ball is not the white one; you're playing Titleist Ones. If this means nothing to you, stay off the course and take a few lessons so you are ready for the next outing.)

If you do know what you're doing out there, the first thing to do is get yourself a proper pair of shoes, which means plastic spikes. As for the rest of your outfit, you can get by without true golf clothes, meaning you can wear a polo shirt, khakis (never shorts), and either a sweater or a windbreaker. Finally, a word of advice if you are very good at golf. Don't embarrass your boss. You don't have to let him win, but if he's got an awful short game, try to put one or two in the woods. And if there's money at stake, and you pocket it, always spring for a round or two at the clubhouse.

TENNIS

Tennis clothing has also benefited from fabric innovation, though the classics—Lacoste shirts, Stan Smith sneakers, etc.—still look smashing.

Sales Meeting... Day

Whether sales conference, sales meeting, or business retreat, it's basically dressing from day to night. In the daytime—business casual (maybe sans socks). In the nighttime—slacks, open neck shirt, and sport coat. In warm weather—linen and cotton rule. And a blazer goes everywhere at these meetings, as it looks good with denim, khakis, and tailored slacks.

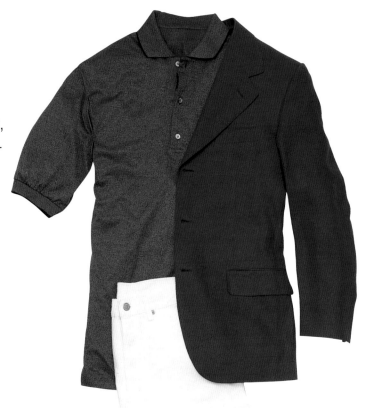

DAYTIME CASUAL

Off-duty, but on. A polo shirt or long-sleeve shirt with a collar, a pair of sporty shoes, a belt, and loafers.

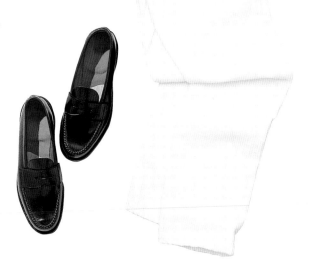

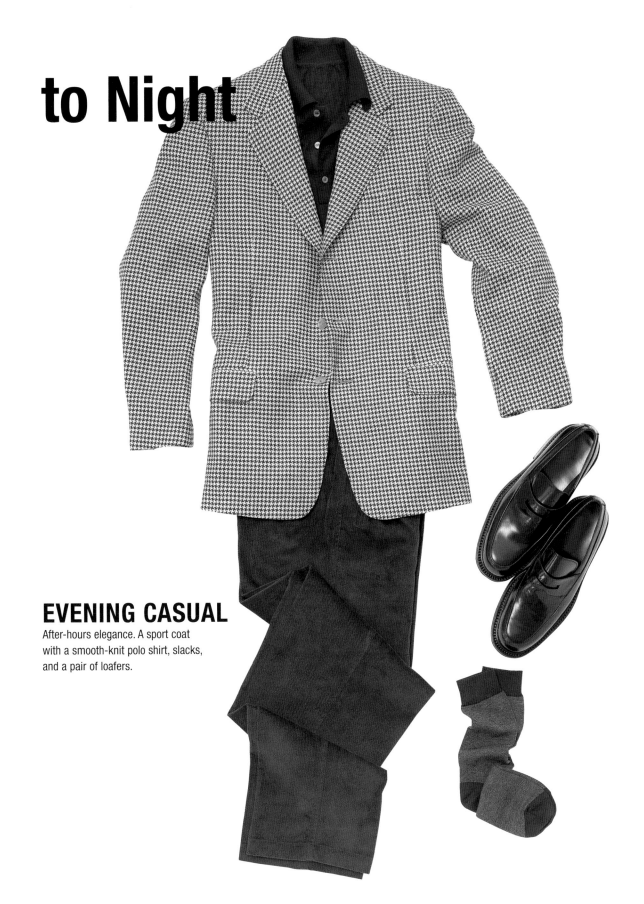

to Night

EVENING CASUAL

After-hours elegance. A sport coat with a smooth-knit polo shirt, slacks, and a pair of loafers.

Healthy Competition

THE TENNIS COURT

DRESS CODE: While tennis whites and a collared shirt are no longer always mandatory, you can never go wrong with them. Keep the shorts at midthigh, and wear clean tennis sneakers and socks.

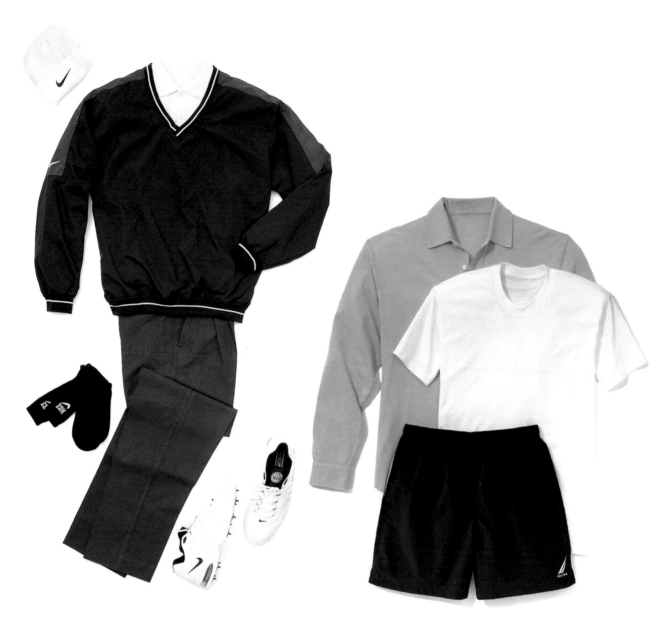

THE GOLF COURSE

DRESS CODE: Pay attention to the course's standards, but in general, long pants, a polo shirt, and golf shoes with soft spikes should be appropriate almost anywhere.

WATER SPORTS

DRESS CODE: Swim trunks should be like shorts and fall somewhere between the thigh and knee. Except when swimming or sun-bathing, wear a clean white T-shirt, a polo shirt, or an oxford button-down.

AVOID: Tight-fitting swimming briefs and extra-long surfer's jams.

Business Entertaining

Business entertaining is one of the hardest working terms in the workplace. Underneath this broad umbrella is everything from bleary-eyed breakfasts with bosses and prospective clients, to box seats at basketball games and opera galas. In general, however, men have an easier time with dressing for these occasions than women, in that a man who dresses appropriately in the daily workplace is usually covered for the drink or dinner date after work. In lieu of changing an outfit, a man can unwrap a new shirt and switch his tie, and go straight from work to most social occasions. The only exceptions are premieres, galas, and black-tie affairs. The line between business suit and black tie continues to blur, but as a rule of thumb the man in the tuxedo at a black-tie optional event feels more comfortable than the guy in the suit fresh from work. Recently the black suit has joined the ranks of the "little black dress" for women. It's dressier than a business suit, but not the "boiled shirt" commitment of a tux. When in doubt, go with the tux.

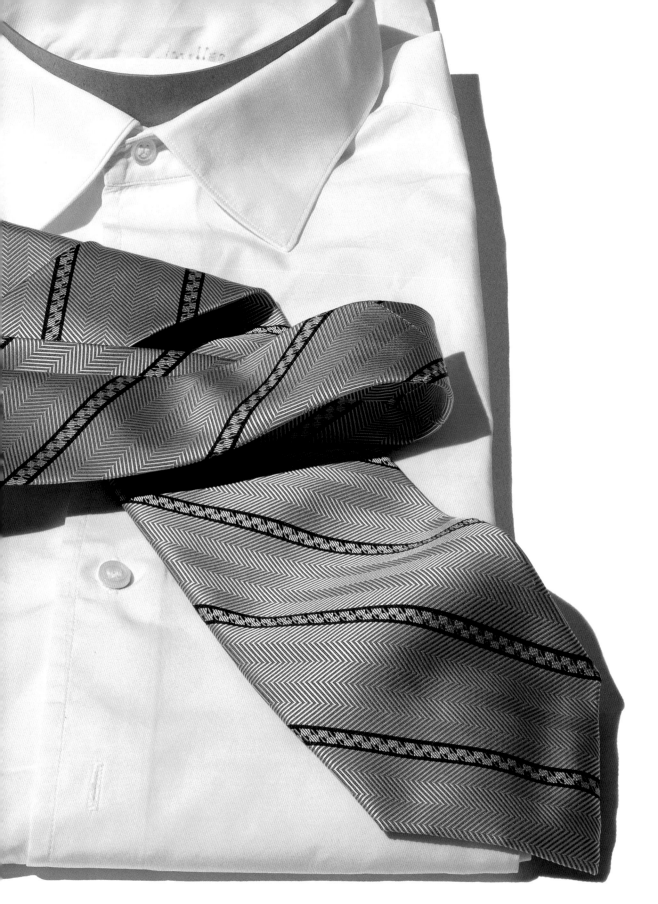

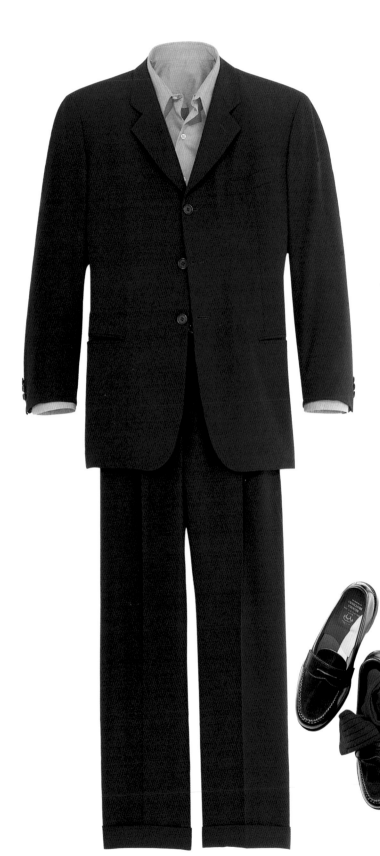

Black

New Classic. Once thought of as the uniform for undertakers and wiseguys, the black suit is now a staple in many men's power wardrobes. There's nothing more sophisticated and urban looking, and also no color that's more slimming.

For day, a black suit can be dressed down with a collared shirt (white, gray, and black work best) and no tie.
FINISHING TOUCHES
To keep the black suit more casual for day, a sportier watch, a simple belt, and a pair of loafers will dress it down slightly.

A.M.

Suit

A black suit may seem too severe for day, but it's right at home at night. It's appropriate for any occasion—from an art opening to a power dinner—and can be dressed up or down accordingly.

The most formal approach to dressing up a black suit is to pair it with a white French cuff shirt and a solid black tie. This outfit can take you out for drinks with the boss after work or to the Academy Awards.
FINISHING TOUCHES
Dress up the suit with a more formal watch, a pair of cuff links for the shirt, an alligator belt (with a silver buckle), and a pair of lace-up shoes (in this case cap-toe oxfords).

P.M.

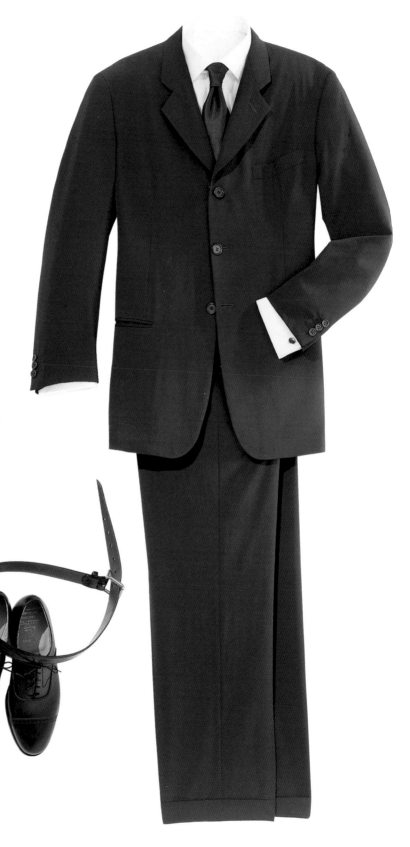

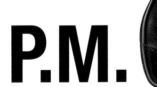

Black Tie

Evening wear is especially kind to men: Put on a well-cut dinner jacket and the appropriate accessories, and suddenly you are Cary Grant or Fred Astaire. While it is hard to get black tie wrong, with a little finesse you can raise it to an art form.

There are three basic styles of tuxedos and all are acceptable. No matter the style, all the lapels should be made of satin or grosgrain, and the bow tie should relate to that material:

Shawl collar. Somewhat rounded lapels.
Notch lapel. Looks like a standard suit jacket.
Peak lapel. Much wider lapel; can be found in single- and double-breasted forms.

Yes, a tuxedo is an expensive investment, but if you consider that it could easily last for five to ten years (assuming you only wear it a few times a year), the cost amortizes out more reasonably.

SHAWL-COLLAR TUXEDO

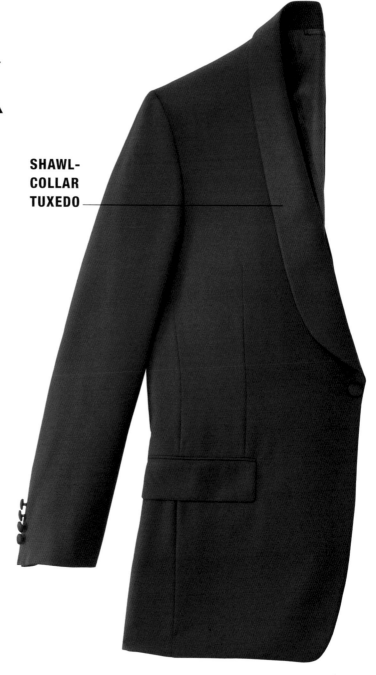

POCKET POWER
A handkerchief in the pocket adds a bit of dash to the tuxedo. To complete the look, a pair of patent leather lace-up shoes is called for—or pumps with satin bows if you're very, very brave.

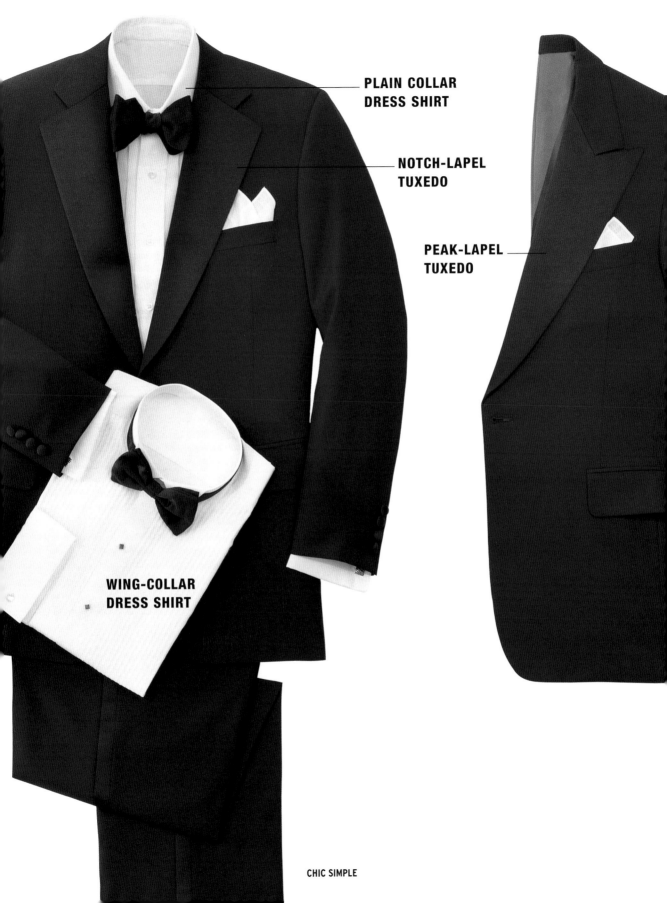

**PLAIN COLLAR
DRESS SHIRT**

**NOTCH-LAPEL
TUXEDO**

**PEAK-LAPEL
TUXEDO**

**WING-COLLAR
DRESS SHIRT**

CHIC SIMPLE

How to: Bow Tie

When it comes to bow ties, the butterfly is the classic shape, and it should always be black. It should also match the cummerbund, which is worn with the pleats facing up.

STEP BY STEP

1. Begin with one end approximately 1^{1}/$_{2}$" below the other and bring the long end up through the center.

2,3. Form a loop with the short end, centering it where the knot will be, and bring the long end over it.

4,5. Form a loop with the long end and push it through the knot behind the front loop.

6. Adjust the ends slowly. This is where the battle of the bow tie is won or lost.

TIP
Practice on your thigh, which is the same circumference as your neck.

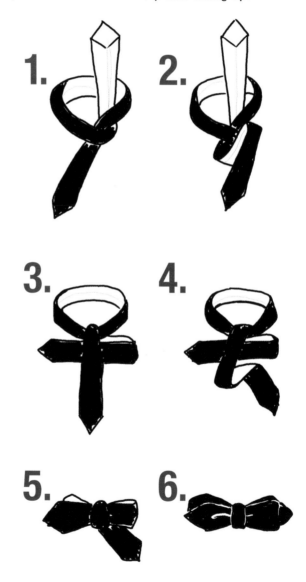

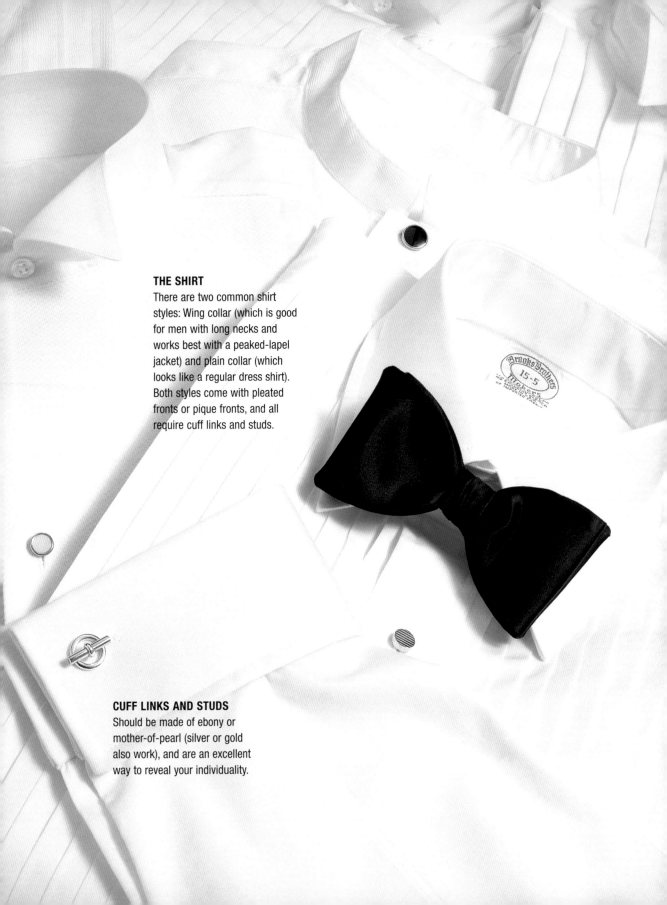

THE SHIRT

There are two common shirt styles: Wing collar (which is good for men with long necks and works best with a peaked-lapel jacket) and plain collar (which looks like a regular dress shirt). Both styles come with pleated fronts or pique fronts, and all require cuff links and studs.

CUFF LINKS AND STUDS

Should be made of ebony or mother-of-pearl (silver or gold also work), and are an excellent way to reveal your individuality.

Dress Smart—A Lifetime Commitment

Despite what many think, clothing is not a luxury: It's a necessity. Look it up. It's nestled there, right in between "food" and "shelter." But how much of it you have and the quality of that clothing is a luxury. Which is why dressing smart, as we have seen, not only reflects the way you look, but also the way you shop for your wardrobe.

To dress smart requires that you know your goals (both professionally and personally), understand your budget, and shop accordingly. But it doesn't end there. Dressing smart is a lifetime commitment. Just as your career takes time and effort, so, too, does building and maintaining a wardrobe. There will be promotions, job changes, moves to new cities, and all will likely require adjustments in your work attire. But you will be ready because you now understand the principles of dressing smart and shopping smart. There is no letting down, because you never know when your next chance to make a first impression will be.

To help you on your path, periodically apply the Chic Simple formula to your life and wardrobe. Assess (your ambitions and your closet), DeJunk (bad habits, worn clothes), ReNew (your commitment to your career and the hard work it will take to get you the things that truly matter to you).

You will come to recognize your wardrobe as one of many tools in the shed. Granted, your clothing is something you need every day, but over time you will hardly come to notice the effort it takes. You will simply be well dressed, and can concentrate on the job at hand.

Nice work.

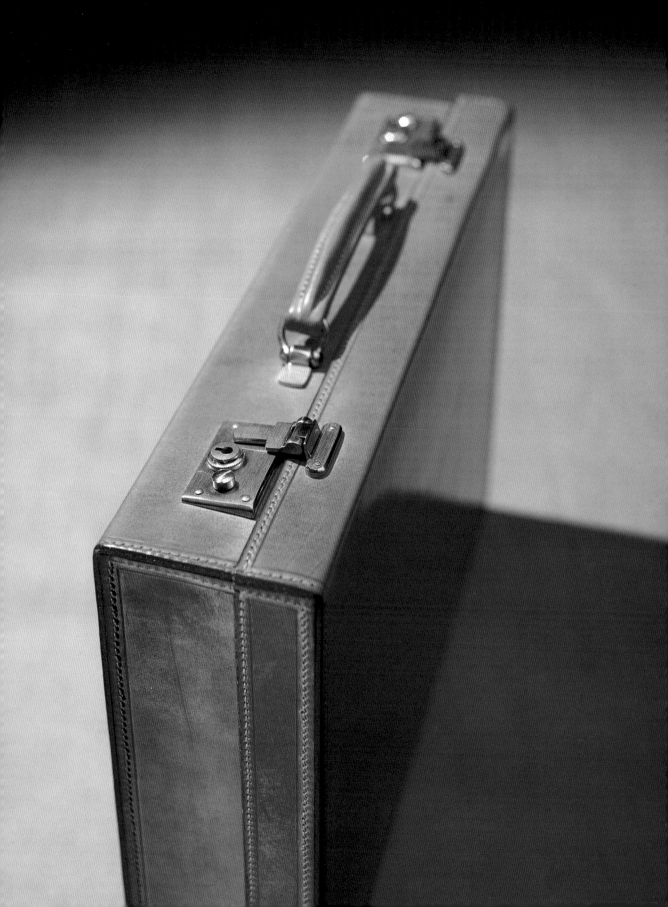

RESOURCES

P 9   shirt—Polo by Ralph Lauren; tie—Tommy Hilfiger; shirt—Hickey Freeman; tie—Paul Stuart; shirt—Hickey Freeman; tie—Robert Talbott Best in Class

P 11   tortoiseshell reading eyeglasses—Liz Claiborne

P 12   tie—Tino Cosmo

P 15   leather suitcase—Peal & Co. Ltd for Brooks Brothers; soft leather briefcase—Bill Auberg

P 20   FROM LEFT silk ties—Garrick Anderson; Gucci; Turnbull & Asser; Hackett; Ermenegildo Zegna; Richel; Hackett; Paul Stuart; Mount Royal; Rooster; Garrick Anderson; Hackett; Ermenegildo Zegna; XMI; Hackett; Brian Bubb; Charvet

P 22   TOP cotton shirt—Garrick Anderson; cuff links—James Robinson; silk knit tie—Hackett; BOTTOM shirt—Alan Flusser; silk tie—Alfred Dunhill

P 24   LEFT pinstripe suit, linen handkerchief, cap-toe shoes—Paul Stuart; spread collar shirt—Paul Stuart "Stuart's Choice"; silk print tie—Brooks Brothers; RIGHT jacket—Bergdorf Goodman; tee—Old Navy; dark rinse jeans—Levi's 501

P 25   LEFT sack suit, belt—Brooks Brothers; oxford cloth button-down, silk knit tie, linen pocket square—Paul Stuart; shoes—J.M. Weston; watch—Holland & Holland RIGHT jacket—DKNY; button-down shirt—J. Crew; linen suit pants—Joseph Abboud; loafers—Gucci; braided leather belt—Dockers; Tank watch—Cartier

P 27   polish—Kiwi; leather cap-toe shoe—Johnston & Murphy; cedar shoe tree—Hold Everything

P 32   suit, shirt, tie, pocket square—Polo by Ralph Lauren

P 35   money clip—Ad Hoc and The Museum of Modern Art

P 38   gold hoop—Monet

P 41   wool suit—Albert Nipon Collection at Lord & Taylor; end-on-end shirt, belt—Brooks Brothers; solid silk tie—J. Crew

P 42   wool suit jacket—Albert Nipon Collection at Lord & Taylor

P 43   wool suit pants—Albert Nipon Collection at Lord & Taylor

P 44   straight point collar shirt—Kenneth Cole

P 45   button down shirt—Brooks Brothers

P 46-47   print tie—Allea Milano at Lord & Taylor; striped tie—Brooks Brothers; solid silk tie—J. Crew; wool suit—see page 41

P 48   leather oxfords with tie—Brooks Brothers

P 49   leather cap-toe oxfords—Brooks Brothers

P 50   embossed leather belt—J.M. Weston; socks—Holland & Holland

P 51   wire frame eyeglasses—Oliver Peoples; plastic frame eyeglasses—Calvin Klein

P 52-53   portfolio—Pina Zangaro San Francisco at Sam Flax; moleskine notebook—Modo et Modo at Sam Flax; leather portfolio—Banana Republic

P 54   stainless steel watch—Indigo by Timex

P 55   leather strap watch—Indigo by Timex

P 56-57   closet items—see all above

P 58   tropical wool suit—Brooks Brothers; oxford cloth shirt, linen handerkerchief—Paul Stuart

P 60   cotton shirt—Polo by Ralph Lauren

P 67   black knit tie—Donna Karan Men

P 75   cashmere coat—Alan Flusser; pinstripe suit, shirt—Joseph Abboud; silk tie—Hermès; silk pocket square, socks—Brooks Brothers; belt—J.M. Weston; cap-toe shoes, cuff knots—Paul Stuart; leather expandable briefcase—T. Anthony

P 76   FROM LEFT wool suit—Albert Nipon Collection at Lord & Taylor; straight point collar shirt—Kenneth Cole; silk tie—J. Crew; wool suit—Albert Nipon Collection at Lord & Taylor; end-on-end shirt, belt with silver buckle—Brooks Brothers; silk tie—J. Crew; worsted wool suit—Kenneth Cole; striped tie, end-on-end shirt, belt with gold buckle—Brooks Brothers; dark gray suit, end-on-end shirt—Brooks Brothers; print tie—Allea Milano at Lord & Taylor

P 77   suit, end-on-end shirt—Brooks Brothers; blue/black print tie—Allea Milano at Lord & Taylor

P 78   wool suit—Albert Nipon Collection at Lord & Taylor; end-on-end shirt, leather belt with silver buckle—Brooks Brothers; solid silk tie—J. Crew

P 79   worsted wool suit—Kenneth Cole; striped tie, end-on-end shirt, leather belt with gold buckle—Brooks Brothers

P 80-81   wool blazer—Nautica at Lord & Taylor

P 82   wool tweed blazer—Lauren Ralph Lauren at Lord & Taylor; trousers, shirt, striped tie with crests—Brooks Brothers

P 83   FROM LEFT worsted wool sport coat—Brooks Brothers; twill sports coat—Lauren Ralph Lauren at Lord & Taylor; wool sport coat—Grant Thomas at Lord & Taylor; wool sport coat—Tommy Hilfiger at Lord & Taylor

P 84   wool tab-front trousers, worsted wool flat-front trousers—Brooks Brothers

P 85   wool flat-front trousers, leather oxfords, flannel tab-front pants—Brooks Brothers; leather loafers—Peal & Co. for Brooks Brothers

P 86   flat-front khakis—Dockers; tab-front khakis—Kenneth Cole; flat-front khakis—Dockers

P 87   thin wale corduroys—Brooks Brothers; wool wide wale corduroys—Banana Republic

P 88   shirts—see pages 89-96

P 89   button-down shirt, striped tie—Brooks Brothers; checked tie—Tommy Hilfiger

P 90   pinpoint shirt—Polo by Ralph Lauren; printed tie—Tommy Hilfiger; navy/gold striped tie—Brooks Brothers

P 91   french blue shirt—Kenneth Cole at Lord & Taylor; silk tie—Claiborne; burgundy/yellow tie—Brooks Brothers

P 92   button-down shirt—Brooks Brothers; Fashion Targets Breast Cancer Tie, paisley tie—Polo by Ralph Lauren

P 93   striped button-down shirt—Brooks Brothers; white/yellow striped tie—Tommy Hilfiger; red silk polka-dot tie—Barneys New York

P 94   pink button-down shirt—Ralph Lauren at Lord & Taylor; green/blue striped tie—Brooks Brothers; yellow/blue print tie—Tommy Hilfiger

P 95   tattersall shirt—Polo by Ralph Lauren; orange/yellow silk tie—Thomas Pink; silk tie—Kenneth Cole

P 96   shirt with french cuffs, french blue silk tie, navy knot cuff link, silver cuff link—Brooks Brothers; red, orange, yellow pattern silk tie—Peter Elliot

P 97   merino wool long-sleeve polo—Brooks Brothers; short-sleeve polo—Barneys New York

P 98-99   cashmere V-neck sweater—Paul Stuart; button-down shirt—Brooks Brothers; tie—Tommy Hilfiger; cashmere vest—Gieves & Hawkes; shirt—Brooks Brothers; blue silk tie—J. Crew

P 100   leather split-toe oxfords—Peal & Co. for Brooks Brothers; blazer—Albert Nipon Collection at Lord & Taylor; cords, socks—Brooks Brothers

P 101   leather penny loafers—Cole Haan; flannel trousers, khakis, socks—Brooks Brothers

P 102   trench with removable lining—Burberry; trench —London Fog; umbrella—Brooks Brothers

P 103   worsted wool suit—Albert Nipon Collection at Lord & Taylor; silk tie, leather gloves—Brooks Brothers; straight point collar shirt—Kenneth Cole at Lord & Taylor; cashmere/silk burgundy scarf—Banana Republic

P 104-105   leather briefcase with gold hardware—Coach; silver pen, money clip—Links of London; leather wallet—Cole Haan; leather date book cover with weekly pocket planner—Exacompta Paris at Sam Flax

P 106-107   closet items—see all above

P 108   leather loafer with silver buckle—Gucci

P 111   cuffs—Bergdorf Goodman Men

P 115   blazer—Ermenegildo Zegna

P 116   sport coat—Alan Flusser

P 117   chambray shirt—Ferrell Reed; white collar chambray shirt—Garrick Anderson

P 119   silk tie—Polo by Ralph Lauren

P 120   suspenders—Polo by Ralph Lauren

P 122   TOP see p 24 left BOTTOM jacket, cuffed trousers—Ermenegildo Zegna; shirt—Polo by Ralph Lauren; sunglasses—Calvin Klein; jack purcell sneakers—Converse; embossed belt—Brooks Brothers; stainless steel watch—Swiss Army

P 123   TOP plaid cashmere suit and vest, cashmere knit tie—Polo by Ralph Lauren; cotton shirt—Ralph Lauren Purple Label; antique silver/enamel "horse & rooster" cuff links—Tender Buttons; watch—Hermès; suede wing-tip shoes—Paul Stuart; socks—Today's Man BOTTOM windowpane wool jacket with vest, shirt, silk tie, gold tie pin, pocket square—Alan Flusser

P 125   silk tie—Gucci

P 127   shirts—see pages 128-132

P 128   wool suit—Ermenegildo Zegna; shirt—Boss Hugo Boss; silk tie—Barneys New York SHIRT/TIE COMBOS CLOCKWISE FROM TOP LEFT straight collar shirt—Hickey Freeman; silk burgundy club tie "Oxxford Shield"—Oxxford Clothes; ecru shirt with french cuffs—Robert Talbott; silk multistripe tie—Ermenegildo Zegna; pink shirt with white spread collar—Robert Talbott; silk pink/black tie—Robert Talbott Best of Class; check spread collar shirt with french cuffs—Robert Talbott; silk and cashmere plaid tie—Robert Talbott Best of Class

P 129   suit—Oxxford Clothes; striped shirt—Boss Hugo Boss; woven tie—Ermenegildo Zegna; SHIRT/TIE COMBOS CLOCKWISE FROM TOP LEFT Egyptian cotton shirt—Joseph Abboud; silk striped tie—Boss Hugo Boss; blue shirt—Hickey Freeman Collection; navy silk woven tie—Paul Stuart; white spread collar shirt—Oxxford Clothes; silk polka-dot tie—Seven Fold; striped shirt—Boss Hugo Boss; silk tie—Oxxford Clothes

P 130   pinstripe suit—Oxxford Clothes; pocket-handkerchief, navy/white knots—Brooks Brothers; chambray shirt with french cuffs and white collar—Paul Stuart; blue print tie—Alan Flusser for Saks Fifth Avenue; SHIRT/TIE COMBOS CLOCKWISE FROM TOP LEFT herringbone moderate spread collar shirt—Paul Stuart; silk tie—Paul Stuart; lavender straight point shirt—Ermenegildo Zegna; silk tie—Ermenegildo Zegna; yellow spread collar shirt with french cuffs—Robert Talbott; silk tie—Robert Talbott; red/pink/gray striped moderate collar shirt—Ermenegildo Zegna; red and gray striped tie—Robert Talbott

P 131 wool suit, straight point collar shirt—Oxxford Clothes; silk tie—Boss Hugo Boss; SHIRT/TIE COMBOS CLOCKWISE FROM TOP LEFT blue striped shirt—Oxxford Clothes; paisley silk tie—Oxxford Clothes; white moderate spread collar shirt with brown/peach plaid—Ermenegildo Zegna; yellow/brown print tie—Zegna; magenta/navy plaid spread collar shirt—Robert Talbott Best of Class; hand-sewn fine silk polka-dot tie—Robert Talbott; striped spread collar shirt with french cuffs—Oxxford Clothes; navy silk tie—Brooks Brothers

P 132 double-breasted wool pinstripe suit, shirt—Paul Stuart; pocket handkerchief—Brooks Brothers; purple silk tie—Oxxford Clothes; SHIRT/TIE COMBOS CLOCKWISE FROM TOP LEFT navy moderate spread collar shirt—Oxxford Clothes; imported silk paisley tie—Robert Talbott; multistripe spread collar shirt—Hickey Freeman; yellow silk tie—Robert Talbott Best of Class; red/white striped shirt with white collar and cuffs—Robert Talbott Best of Class; black/white polka-dot tie—Seven Fold; yellow spread collar shirt—Robert Talbott; navy silk tie—Robert Talbott Best of Class

P 133 check hidden snap button shirt, silk patterned tie—Giorgio Armani Classico; cotton check "custom-made" shirt—AC by Ascot Chang

P 134-135 wool blazer—Giorgio Armani; straight point collar shirt—Brooks Brothers; thin stripe silk tie—Banana Republic; wool doublebreasted blazer—Paul Stuart; spread collar shirt—Brooks Brothers; silk blend striped tie—Robert Talbott; linen blazer—Ralph Lauren Purple Label; straight point collar shirt—Kenneth Cole; silk novelty tie—Brooks Brothers

P 136-137 plaid moderate spread collar shirt, striped tie—Robert Talbott Estate; white shirt with large checks—Thomas Pink; tie—Oxxford Clothes; striped shirt—Boss Hugo Boss; tie—Joseph Abboud; lavender shirt—Paul Stuart; tie—Joseph Abboud; blue shirt—Joseph Abboud; Tie—Robert Talbott Estate; striped shirt—Paul Stuart; tie—Joseph Abboud; black snap button-down shirt—Polo by Ralph Lauren

P 138 leather blazer—Joseph Abboud; cashmere turtleneck, trousers—Oxxford Clothes

P 139 wool houndstooth/check sport coat—Paul Stuart; tattersall spread collar shirt with french cuffs—Robert Talbott Estate; striped tie—Robert Talbott Best of Class; gold enamel cuff links—Robert Talbott; dress pants—Joseph Abboud

P 140 linen sport coat, linen pants—Polo by Ralph Lauren; moderate spread collar shirt—Ermenegildo Zegna; silk plaid tie—Joseph Abboud; wool pleated pants—Hickey Freeman

P 141 houndstooth sport coat—Grant Thomas at Lord & Taylor; merino wool long-sleeve sweater, worsted wool flat-front pants—Brooks Brothers; multistripe straight collar shirt, silk tie—Giorgio Armani Classico; wide wale corduroys—Banana Republic

P 142 herringbone super 100s wool sport coat, wool trousers—Oxxford Clothes; moderate spread collar shirt, cashmere tie—Robert Talbott Best of Class; wool trousers—Brooks Brothers

P 143 moleskin sports coat—Oxxford Clothes; moderate spread collar shirt—Robert Talbott Best of Class; silk/wool blend tie—Ermenegildo Zegna; boot cut jeans—Levi's; cotton blend corduroys—Brooks Brothers

P 144-145 leather loafers with buckle—Gucci; leather tassel loafers, patent leather loafers, leather cap-

toe oxfords, suede shoes—Brooks Brothers

P 146-147 leather briefcase with gold hardware—T. Anthony; sterling silver watch casing with leather wristband—IWC Schaffhausen; hand-crafted alligator belt—Coach; sterling silver etched belt buckle, sterling silver cuff links with etching, handkerchief—Brooks Brothers; blue-edged handkerchief, maroon-edged handkerchief—Paul Stuart

P 148 silk/cashmere reversible scarf—Salvatore Ferragamo; coat—Polo by Ralph Lauren

P 149 norfolk jacket—Holland & Holland

P 150-151 closet items—see all above

P 152 vertical wardrobe—Innovation Wardrobe

P 159 CLOCKWISE FROM LEFT cotton T-shirts—The Gap; river shorts—Patagonia; travel gear—personal collection of JS; leather loafers—Cole-Haan; leather duffel bag—Ghurka; cashmere sweater—Paul Stuart; 501 jeans—Levi Strauss & Co.; tie case—Bottega Veneta; silk tie—Alan Flusser; silk knit tie—Barneys; leather Dopp Kit—Ghurka; sneakers—Nike

P 160 nylon computer bag/carry-on—Tumi; soft garment bag—Innovation Luggage

P 161 nylon wheelie—Tumi; Dopp Kit case—T. Anthony

P 162 soft carry-on—Hartmann Luggage-E. Vincent Luggage; metal luggage—Zero Halliburton-Bettingers

P 164 vertical luggage—Innovation Luggage (clothing throughout book)

P 165 shirts FROM TOP Polo; Vestimenta; Alan Flusser; Brooks Brothers; tie, tie case—private collection; shoes, socks—Dockers

P 166 wool/cashmere jacket—Saks Fifth Avenue; cashmere turtleneck, wool trousers—Brooks Brothers; shoes—J. M. Weston; knit tie—Polo; leather belt, socks—Dockers; loafers—Brooks Brothers

P 167 wool trousers—A/X; cashmere jacket—Polo; cashmere V-neck pullover—J. Crew; flat-front khaki pants—Dockers

P 171 silver cocktail shaker—Pedrini; martini glass—Crate & Barrel

P 174 linen jacket—Bergdorf Goodman; golf shirt—Bobby Jones; cotton 501 jeans—Levi Strauss & Co.; suede shoes—Cole-Haan

P 175 houndstooth blazer—Ermenegildo Zegna; cashmere polo—Malo; corduroy pants—Joseph Abboud; polished calf loafers—Prada; socks—Today's Man; sunglasses—Ray•Ban; embossed belt—Trafalgar; vintage watch—International Watch Co.

P 176 cotton polo shirt—Lacoste

P 177 long-sleeve polo, swim trunks—Nautica; crewneck T-shirt—Brooks Brothers; hat, golf shirt, pullover, charcoal shadow plaid golf pants, socks, white airmax 2 leather golf shoes—Nike

P 178-179 shirt—The Shirt Store; silk tie—Ferrell Reed

P 180 suit—Giorgio Armani; shirt—Barneys New York; watch—Swiss Army; leather belt—Banana Republic; leather loafer with silver buckle—Gucci

P 181 suit—Giorgio Armani; shirt—Polo; silk tie—Boss Hugo Boss; cuff links—Brooks Brothers; leather belt—Trafalgar; leather shoes—Cole-Haan

P 182 classic 110's wool shawl collar tuxedo jacket—Hickey Freeman

P 183 wool one-button notch collar tuxedo with satin notch lapel, silk bow tie—Paul Stuart; handkerchiefs—Brooks Brothers; silver/enamel cuff links—Links of London; tuxedo shirt with wing collar—Hickey Freeman; vintage studs—Links

of London; silk bow tie—Boss Hugo Boss; super 100 wool peak lapel tuxedo jacket—Paul Stuart

P 185 CLOCKWISE FROM LEFT tuxedo shirt with tucked bib—Paul Stuart; pleat-front tuxedo shirt with wing collar—Brooks Brothers; pleat-front tuxedo shirt with wing collar—Polo by Ralph Lauren; tuxedo shirt with band collar—Donna Karan; pleat-front tuxedo shirt—Brooks Brothers; silk bow tie—Barneys New York; gold shirt studs—Tiffany; silver/gold cuff links—Hermès; tuxedo shirt with pique bib and wing collar, 14-karat gold cuff links—Paul Stuart

P 187 briefcase—T. Anthony

QUOTES

P 8 John T. Molloy, *New Dress for Success* (Warner, 1988)

P 15 Mark Twain, from *The Forbes Book of Business Quotations*, Ted Goodman (Black Dog & Leventhal Publishers, Inc., 1997)

P 17 Malcolm Forbes, from *The Quotable Executive*, John Woods (McGraw-Hill, 2000)

P 18 Michael Korda, *Power! How to Get It, How to Use It* (Random House, 1975)

P 23 Gerald J. Simmons, from *The Forbes Book of Business Quotations*, Ted Goodman (Black Dog & Leventhal Publishers, Inc., 1997)

P 31 Simon Doonan, *The New York Observer*, April 15, 2002

P 33 Tom Masson, from *The Quotable Executive*, John Woods (McGraw-Hill, 2000)

P 37, 40 Roger Ailes, *You Are the Message* (Doubleday & Co., 1996)

P 61 Craig Pogson, *Maître d' at Orsay*

P 63 Gertrude Stein, "What Is English Literature," 1934 from *The New York Public Library Book of 20th Century American Quotations*, Ed. Stephen Donadio, Joan Smith, Susan Mesner, Rebecca Davidson (Warner, 1992)

P 64 Roland Young, from *The Forbes Book of Business Quotations*, Ted Goodman (Black Dog & Leventhal Publishers, Inc., 1997)

P 65 Mae West, from *The Art of Looking Sideways*, Alan Fletcher (Phaidon Press Limited, 2001)

P 66 French management saying, from *The Forbes Book of Business Quotations*, Ted Goodman (Black Dog & Leventhal Publishers, Inc., 1997)

P 70 Joseph Heller, *Catch-22* (Simon & Schuster, 1961)

P 71 J. Pierpont Morgan, from *The Quotable Executive*, John Woods (McGraw-Hill, 2000)

P 74 Henry Ford, from *The New York Public Library Book of 20th Century American Quotations*, Stephen Donadio, et al. (Warner, 1992)

P 110 Anonymous, from *The International Thesaurus of Quotations, Revised and Updated* (HarperPerennial, 1996)

P 126 Jerry Rubin, *Growing (Up) at Thirty-Seven* (M. Evans & Co., 1976)

P 155 Carol Channing, from *Simpson's Contemporary Quotations, Revised Edition*, James Simpson (HarperCollins, 1997)

P 158 Woody Allen, from *The New York Public Library Book of 20th Century American Quotations*, Ed. Stephen Donadio, Joan Smith, Susan Mesner, Rebecca Davidson (Warner, 1992)

P 170 George Santayana, *Interpretations of Poetry and Religion (1900)*, from *The International Thesaurus of Quotations, Revised and Updated* (HarperPerennial, 1996)

P 192 Michael Korda, *Power! How to Get It, How to Use It* (Random House, 1975)

PHOTOGRAPHY BY DAVID BASHAW EXCEPT:

James Wojick: 20 ties; 22 shirts/ties; 32 suit; 35 clip; 36 notepad; 38 hoop; 60 shirt; 85 tie; 44 cuffs; 115 jacket; 116 jacket; 117 shirts; 119 tie; 120 suspenders; 125 tie; 148 coat; 152 suitcase; 160 garment bag; 161 dopp kit; 162 suitcases; 164 packing; 164 shirts, case; 166-167 clothes; 169 qtips; 178 shirt/tie; 187 case **José Picayo:** 148 scarf **Dana Gallagher:** 10 pencil **Robert Tardio:** 103 suit (right) **ILLUSTRATIONS** Eric Hanson: globe **Ruth Ansel:** Kim and jeff

DEDICATION

With love to my children, Glenna and Carolyn, who make my world rich and big, to my very chic simple mother, Evelyn Johnson, and to my sisters, Susan Banta and Jill Johnson, who live life with adventure and style—Kim

None of this could have happened without Jane's support and patience along with the entire army of children we share from Stef, to Dylan, Bradley and Morgan. Thanks, boys, for your love and support. Also great appreciation to Rob and Kinney, Peter, Victor and Max (always forget who is in ascension) and Tim and Taylor for the friendship and love they all have shared with the guys—Jeff

ACKNOWLEDGMENTS

Lord & Taylor, Brooks Brothers, Talbots, Ralph Lauren, Nordstrom; Banana Republic, John Molloy—*Dress for Success*; Caterine Milinaire—*Cheap Chic*

INVALUABLE RESOURCES

Caryn Karmatz Rudy, Molly Chehak, Binky Urban, Ruth Ansel, Mitchell Rosenbaum, Seth Bogner, Ali, Eugenia Fickens, Henry at Union Square Cafe, Steve at Michaels, Gregory Giangrande

CHIC SIMPLE STAFF

Partners Kim & Jeff
President Jim Winters
Style Consultant Laurie Bliss
Associate Style Editor Samantha Schoengold
Assistant Style Editor Marika Horacek
Production Director Andrea Weinreb
Office Manager Doug Moe

COMMUNICATIONS

Hi, good to be talking book talk again. It's been a couple of years since our last Chic Simple book. We weren't on vacation, just growing the company. But as we said in the opening letter, we felt there was a need to address the changing landscape of dressing in today's current workplace, and books still work best. We still have our web site up, www.chicsimple.com, which we get annoyed at because it is always lagging behind what we are doing—the Internet is like a public in-box of things constantly needing attention. It's good hearing from all of you, even the woman from Paris who came up to us as we were eating fish tacos at Club Havana (it's just hard to talk with your mouth full). And it made us so happy to hear from Remo the other day; let's hear it for Australia. The big news is we moved out of the SoHo loft to an office overlooking Union Square. There is something very special in being suspended over trees in New York City. As usual you can write or e-mail or fax us at the office:

Chic Simple
200 Park Avenue South
New York, New York 10003
Fax: 212-473-0204
www.chicsimple.com

A NOTE ON THE TYPE

Why do we even comment on the type we use? Well, we like type and with the advent of computers everyone has tried his or her hand on the use of fonts and playing with size and styles. Who hasn't blown up type or played with **bold** and *italic*? Chic Simple has always tried to use type as an element of design and also entertainment—which occasionally appears to annoy people. For many books we used New Baskerville (a serif typeface) for what is called the body copy, and for captions and factoids the typeface Futura (sans serif) was utilized. The body copy of the two new Chic Simple titles is set in Minion while the captions and image guide information is in a sans-serif called Helvetica Neue. **MINION** was created by Robert Slimbach; it's a classical and very readable type we feel makes you feel like you are with an old friend, which is what a book should be about. What's nice about it is its aesthetic—a page looks pretty and somehow elegant wearing it—while it's still readable, a nice functional quality in a typeface. Helvetica is the type of "the NEW" and like all things of the "new" it was createded in the 60s. It was developed in 1961 by the German foundry D. Stempel AG and was originally named "Neue Haas Grotesk." We guess someone in the marketing department mentioned that to have your customers constantly refering to your product as grotesque might not be a brilliant move, so the name Helvetica came into being. Smart move: Helvetica has become the most popular typeface in the world. The version used in the two new books is called **HELVETICA NEUE**, which is a redrawn version of Helvetica with better uniformity between the different weights. Essentially it means that the different sizes and bold appearances are more balanced. We're sure this is way more information than you could possibly desire, but have you ever known us not to beat a subject to death?

SEPARATION AND FILM BY

Butler & Tanner Limited
Frome, England

PRINTED AND BOUND BY

Butler & Tanner Limited
Frome, England

HARDWARE

It used to be fun to walk around the office as Chic Simple was growing and list all the cool equipment that was being used to create the books. The first books were done with state-of-the-art Apple Macintosh Quad 700's. Ah those were the days. Remember how if the files were too big instead of a photo that awful message would come up in a field of gray, NOT ENOUGH MEMORY? And for accessing the Internet there was a noble Supra Modem: Download time was measured in days. Today it's just overwhelming: We have old rugged stealth Macintosh G-3's, fancy Macintosh G-4's with attitude, iMacs running around the halls misbehaving, and the occasional slightly disapproving PC. There are hubs, networks scanners, and a growing battery of printers whose sole purpose is to sit around in the afternoon and swig toner. Everyone seems to be IM-ing online and we still don't understand what happened between T-1 and T-3 lines; did we just miss T-2s? Also, where does old equipment go? It seems to just disappear. Is it like elephants? Is there somewhere near Santa Cruz or San Jose a field full of old Syquest drives in retirement? Anyway, most of our storage is devoted to MP-3s which is a segue into...

MUSICWARE

Wilco (*Summerteeth*), Morphine (*Good*), St. Germain (*Tourist*), Air (*Moon Safari*), Michael Bloomfield (*Don't Say That I Ain't Your Man*), Eric Clapton & B.B. King (*Riding with the King*), Van Morrison (*Philosopher's Stone*), Arturo Delmon/Nathaniel Rosen (*Music for a Glass Bead Game*), Philp Glass (*Dancepieces*), Sir Neville Marriner (*Mozart Wind Concerti*), Lucinda Williams (*Essence*), The Roches (*Zero Church*), Various Artists (*WFUV-City Folk Live*), Ja Rule (*Pain Is Love*), Various Artists (*Le Flow*), Various Artists (*Jackson Pollock Jazz*), Charles Lloyd (*Voices in the Night*), Charlie Haden (*Nocturne*), Chet Baker (*Sentimental in Paris*), Django Reinhart & Stephane Grappelli (*Swing from Paris*), Louis Armstrong (*Hot Fives & Sevens*), Oscar Peterson (*Plays Count Basie*), Roy Hargrove (*Moment to Moment*), Sarah Vaughan (*The Complete Mercury*), Badly Drawn Boy (*The Hour of Bewilderbeast*), Bruce Springsteen (*Bootleg Philadelphia Concert*—Thank you George), U2 (*Beautiful Day*), Harmonia Ensemble (*Fellini-L'Uomo del Sogni*), Anne Sofie von Otter & Elvis Costello (*For the Stars*), Frank Sinatra (*Songs for Swinging Lovers*), Paolo Conte (*The Best of*), Tom Waits (*Beautiful Maladies*), Bob Marley (*Songs of Freedom-Disc 4*), Mercedes Sosa (*30 Años*), Omara Portuondo (*Omara Portuondo*), Charles Aznavour (*Greatest Golden Hits*), June Tabor (*Against the Streams*), Bryan Ferry (*As Time Goes By*), Jussi Bjoerling (*The Pearl Fishers Duet*), June Monheit (*Never Never Land*), Van Morrison with George Fame & Friends (*How Long Has This Been Going On*), Wong Kar-wai (*In the Mood for Love*), Bebel Gilberto (*Tanto Tempo*), Cesaria Evora (*Cafe Atlantico*), Etta James (*Blue Gardenia*), Joe Henderson (*Lush Life*), Bob Dylan (*Love and Theft*), Leonard Cohen (*Ten New Songs*). None of the books could ever have made it through the dark empty nights of flowing copy into pages without the steadfast beacon of **PIG** radio (KPIG to the uninitiated) beaming its message of a better world through pick'n and sing'n from its golden home on the shores of Freedom county to the dark twisted urban canyon lands of our New York offices. Thank you, PIG.
jeff and Kim

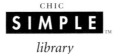

CHIC
SIMPLE™
library

"All life is a game of power. The object of the game is simple enough: to know what you want and get it."

MICHAEL KORDA, *Power!*